Populism and the Politicization of the COVID-19 Crisis in Europe

Giuliano Bobba · Nicolas Hubé
Editors

Populism and the Politicization of the COVID-19 Crisis in Europe

palgrave
macmillan

Editors
Giuliano Bobba
Department of Cultures, Politics
and Society—Collegio Carlo Alberto
University of Turin
Turin, Italy

Nicolas Hubé
Centre for Research on Mediations
(CREM)
University of Lorraine
Metz, France

ISBN 978-3-030-66010-9 ISBN 978-3-030-66011-6 (eBook)
https://doi.org/10.1007/978-3-030-66011-6

This Palgrave Macmillan imprint is published by the registered company Springer Nature Switzerland AG
The registered company address is: Gewerbestrasse 11, 6330 Cham, Switzerland

Acknowledgments

This work was supported by the European Union's Horizon 2020 research and innovation programme under grant agreement No. 822590 (Democratic Efficacy and the Varieties of Populism in Europe).

Contents

Contributors

Martin Baloge Centre for Research on Mediations (CREM), University of Lorraine, Metz, France

Márton Bene Centre for Social Sciences, Budapest, Hungary

Arturo Bertero Department of Cultures, Politics and Society, University of Turin, Turin, Italy

Giuliano Bobba Department of Cultures, Politics and Society—Collegio Carlo Alberto, University of Turin, Turin, Italy

Zsolt Boda Centre for Social Sciences, Budapest, Hungary

Ondřej Císař Charles University, Prague, Czechia

Nicolas Hubé Centre for Research on Mediations (CREM), University of Lorraine, Metz, France

Bogdan Ianosev Glasgow Caledonian University, Glasgow, Scotland, UK

Michal Kubát Charles University, Prague, Czechia

Oliver W. Lembcke Ruhr-University Bochum, Bochum, Germany

Artur Lipiński Adam Mickiewicz University, Poznań, Poland

Jaume Magre Universitat de Barcelona and Fundació Carles Pi i Sunyer, Barcelona, Spain

Lluís Medir Universitat de Barcelona, Barcelona, Spain

Esther Pano Universitat de Barcelona and Fundació Carles Pi i Sunyer, Barcelona, Spain

Osman Sahin Glasgow Caledonian University, Glasgow, Scotland, UK

Antonella Seddone Department of Cultures, Politics and Society, University of Turin, Turin, Italy

Abbreviations

Translated Name of the Party	*Original Name of the Party*	*Acronym*
United Kingdom		
United Kingdom Independence Party	United Kingdom Independence Party	UKIP
Brexit Party	Brexit Party	Brexit Party
Spain		
Spanish Socialist Workers' Party	Partido Socialista Obrero Español	PSOE
People's Party	Partido Popular	PP
VOX	VOX	VOX
United We Can	Unidas Podemos	UP
Citizens	Ciudadanos	C's
Italy		
Go Italy	Forza Italia	FI
Brothers of Italy	Fratelli d'Italia	FdI
League	Lega	Lega
Five Star Movement	Movimento 5 Stelle	M5S
Democratic Party	Partito Democratico	PD
France		
National Rally	Rassemblement National	RN
Indomitable France	La France Insoumise	LFI
The Republic on the Move	La République en Marche	LREM
MODEM	MODEM	MODEM
Democrats and Independants' Union	Union des Démocrates et Indépendants	UDI

(continued)

(continued)

Translated Name of the Party	*Original Name of the Party*	*Acronym*
Socialist Party	Parti Socialiste	PS
Greens	Les Verts	EELV
The Republicans	Les Républicains	LR
Germany		
Alternative for Germany	Alternative für Deutschland	AfD
Federal Minister of Health	Bundesministerium für Gesundheit	BMG
Christian Democratic Union	Christlich Demokratische Union Deutschlands	CDU
Christian Social Union in Bavaria	Christlich-Soziale Union in Bayern	CSU
Liberal Democratic Party	Freie Demokratische Partei	F.D.P.
Green Party	Bündnis 90/Die Grünen	Grüne
The Left Party	Die Linke	Linke
Robert Koch Institute	Robert Koch Institut	RKI
Social Democratic Party	Sozialdemokratische Partei Deutschlands	SPD
Hungary		
Fidesz	Fidesz	Fidesz
Christian Democratic People's Party	Kereszténydemokrata Néppárt	KDNP
Hungarian Socialist Party	Magyar Szocialista Párt	MSZP
For a Better Hungary	Jobbik Magyarországért Mozgalom	Jobbik
Democratic Coalition	Demokratikus Koalíció	DK
Another Politics Is Possible	Lehet Más a Politika	LMP
Momentum	Momentum	Momentum
Dialogue	Párbeszéd	P
Czech Republic		
ANO 2011	ANO 2011	ANO
Freedom and Direct Democracy	Svoboda a přímá demokracie	SPD
Communist Party of Bohemia and Moravia	Komunistická strana Čech a Moravy	KSČM
Poland		
Law and Justice	Prawo i Sprawiedliwość	PiS
Confederation 'Freedom and Independence'	Konfederacja 'Wolność i Niepodległość'	Confederation
Civic Platform	Platforma Obywatelska	PO
Polish People's Party	Polskie Stronnictwo Ludowe	PSL
Democratic Left Alliance	Sojusz Lewicy Demokratycznej	SLD

List of Figures

Chapter 9

Chapter 10

List of Tables

Chapter 6

Chapter 7

Chapter 8

Chapter 9

Chapter 10

CHAPTER 1

COVID-19 and Populism: A Sui Generis Crisis

Giuliano Bobba and Nicolas Hubé

1 Introduction

Although the debate about the link between crises and populism is a lengthy one, several authors agree that alleged crisis situations are a precondition for the emergence of populist mobilization. Or at least that they can favour it. While the impact of COVID-19 has not been the same in countries around the world, in many of them this pandemic has been the biggest health and, in its aftermath, economic crisis since World War II. Despite the peculiar nature of this crisis, however, it is not obvious how populists may benefit from it. Like other catastrophes or natural events, COVID-19 is hard to politicize, that is, to become an arena of political confrontation among parties with the traditional divides

G. Bobba (✉)
Department of Cultures, Politics and Society—Collegio Carlo Alberto,
University of Turin, Turin, Italy
e-mail: giuliano.bobba@unito.it

N. Hubé
Centre for Research on Mediations (CREM),
University of Lorraine, Metz, France
e-mail: nicolas.hube@univ-lorraine.fr

G. Bobba and N. Hubé (eds.), *Populism and the Politicization of the COVID-19 Crisis in Europe*,
https://doi.org/10.1007/978-3-030-66011-6_1

(us vs. others; elites vs. people), at least in its initial stage. This crisis has popped up without having been triggered by populists as a consequence of the failure of the elite, migrants, etc. (Moffitt 2015). The chapter will provide a framework of analysis, discussing the literature on crises and populism from a theoretical perspective and in the light of the concept of politicization. It will then offer an overview of the main contents of the book.

2 Crisis and Populism

Populism is an 'essentially contested concept' (Mudde and Rovira Kaltwasser 2017) and there is a lengthy debate on its definition and whether it can be considered as an ideology (Mudde 2004, 2007; Taggart 2000), a communication style (de Vreese et al. 2018; Aalberg et al. 2017; Jagers and Walgrave 2007; Moffitt 2016) or a political strategy (Weyland 2001; Roberts 1995). Nevertheless, scholars generally agree on a minimum definition of populism: the juxtaposition of the 'good people' with a series of 'bad elites' and disturbing out-groups (notable exceptions include Müller 2016 and Urbinati 2019). Populists in Western democracies present themselves as the 'real' democrats committed to explaining to the people 'what went wrong, who is to blame, and what is to be done to reverse the situation' (Betz and Johnson 2004: 323). Democracy should be an 'expression of the *volonté générale* (general will) of the people' (Mudde 2004: 544); instead, it has been usurped by 'the elites' who are to blame for all the major problems affecting 'the people'. The positive valuation of 'the people' is thus combined with the denigration of their enemies, namely 'the elites' who are accused of being arrogant, corrupt and more generally of acting against 'the people' (Canovan 1999: 5), and out-groups (migrants, LGBT, etc.), accused of othering the essential nature of the 'real people'.

Similarly, the concept of the crisis has been widely associated with populism, although there is some debate about the nature of the link between the two phenomena. 'Crisis' is a term with a long history in the field of political philosophy and political science (Koselleck 2006). From different perspectives, classical theorists such as Karl Marx (1981), Antonio Gramsci (1971) and Jürgen Habermas (1975) considered the crisis as a critical conjuncture undermining State authority and offering an opportunity for change. A crisis is not only an objective phenomenon; it also needs to be subjectively perceived as such and/or discursively pushed to the forefront by political actors.

According to Colin Hay (1999: 317), while the concept of the crisis is ubiquitous within social and political thought, it remains one of the most 'elusive, imprecise and generally unspecified concepts within the theoretician's armoury'. In the literature, the concept of crisis is used to name mutually incompatible conditions, processes and properties. For example, crises are generally considered temporary, but they can also be permanent; they are a one-off deviation from the natural course of events, but they can also be cyclical; normally they have a solution, but they can also be unsolvable. Hay addresses this gap by making an analytical distinction between the *objective* and *subjective* components of crises (see also Habermas 1975). On the one hand, contradictions can intentionally be addressed by an agent through a decisive or inconclusive intervention (objective component). On the other hand, the same contradictions can be subjectively perceived as such or remain publicly unacknowledged. The combination of these two components results in a typology in which the crisis is only one of the different types of possible systemic contradictions and responses.

A *crisis* is a moment in which systemic contradictions (i.e. failures) are widely perceived as salient in the political, cultural or ideological spheres and decisive interventions and structural transformations are implemented. A political crisis occurs when the common rationalities in solving the problem are blurred and when agents appear to be overwhelmed in handling the facts in all areas of the crisis. The other names for it are *failure*, *tipping point* and *catastrophic equilibrium*. *Failure* is an accumulation of unresolved systemic contradictions and the dysfunctional symptoms they generate, regardless of individuals' perception or awareness. It provides the 'structural preconditions for perceived crisis; the necessary but insufficient conditions' for a crisis (Hay 1999: 324). A *tipping point* is a moment at which an intervention made unintentionally, in a situation of unperceived systemic contradictions, subsequently 'proves to be decisive in terms of the transformation of the system in question' (325). Finally, *catastrophic equilibrium* (Gramsci 1971: 276) refers to a situation in which symptoms of systemic contradictions are commonly recognized as a wider problem, even in the absence of mobilization and decisive intervention.

The COVID-19 pandemic led European countries to a peculiar crisis situation where neither national healthcare systems nor the World Health

Organization were able to predict or control the risk, and where the medical sciences were unable to face the pandemic effectively or rationally. The nature of the crisis does not fit in with the common problem-solving schemes of an economic or migration crisis and this is the main difference with the last decade of 'crisis-ridden Europe' in which populists have grown, sometimes playing an active role (Kriesi and Pappas 2015: 303; see also Trenz et al. 2015).

3 Role of Crisis in Contemporary Populism

In this paragraph, we need to disentangle the literature on crises and that on populism in order to better understand the role of crises in the rise of populism and the role of populists in the rise of crises. The role of crises in the contemporary populist literature is disputed. While it is quite common to find references to crises in the populist literature, studies devoted to this connection are rare and it remains in many respects under-theorized: the term is normally used in a vague manner, with no definition provided. Nevertheless, except for a few authors who have contested any link between crises and populism (i.e. Knight 1998; Arditi 2007), scholars addressing this topic generally fall into two broad categories: those who state that there is a direct connection between the existence of a crisis and the rise of populism, and those who are less sure about a causal link between these two processes.

Ernesto Laclau (1977, 2005) is certainly one of the first scholars link the rise of populism to crises. According to Laclau (1977: 175), 'the emergence of populism is historically linked to a crisis of the dominant ideological discourse, which in turn is part of a more general social crisis'. In other words, populism simply cannot emerge without a political crisis, which is considered a 'necessary precondition for populism' (2005: 177). A crisis of representation in particular is what allows populists to emerge and succeed. Several authors agree that this particular kind of political crisis is at the root of any populist mobilization (see Canovan 1999; Roberts 1995, 2015; Kriesi 2015; Mouffe 2005). Among them, Hanspeter Kriesi (2015) links the current rise of populists in Europe to long-term trends in political representation. As party democracy weakens, 'the opportunities for populist protest clearly increases' (Mair 2002: 88). This process is even more evident in the light of the new 'integration-demarcation' divide caused by the process of globalization (Kriesi et al. 2006, 2012). Party democracy is facing new challenges, since 'divide theory meets Europe's crises' (Hooghe and Marks 2017), and Euroscepticism, like populism, is becoming more mainstream (Conti 2018). In Kriesi's words, 'the lack of responsiveness of established parties to the plight of the 'globalization losers' provided a chance for their mobilization by the new populist right parties (2015: 178).

Focusing on Latin American populism, Kenneth Roberts (1995, 2015) similarly argues that weak political institutions and crises of representation trigger different types of populist mobilization in the region: top-down or plebiscitary mobilizations (i.e. Hugo Chavez in Venezuela) coexist with bottom-up or participatory mobilizations (i.e. Evo Morales in Bolivia). Crises could of course have other natures besides political representation. Kurt Weyland (1999: 395) argued that crises of economic neoliberalism triggered the emergence of 'neoliberal populism' in Latin America, with specific reference to Carlos Menem in Argentina, Fernando Collor in Brazil and Alberto Fujimori in Peru. While Kriesi (2015) argues that a crisis of representation is 'the basic condition' for the rise of populism, an economic crisis is considered as a facilitating condition. In the last few years, several authors have interpreted the performance of populist parties as linked to the Great Recession and the European debt crisis (Kriesi and Pappas 2015; Kneuer 2019), while others have pointed to the role of migrant and refugee crises (Brubaker 2017; Stojarová 2018). For these authors, some kind of political and economic crisis is a necessary precondition—and the main explanation—for the emergence of populism.

A second strand of literature is, however, more cautious about the link between crises and populism. As an advocate of the ideological approach, Mudde (2007) states that the concept of crisis is used too vaguely to have a heuristic value. While this link seems to be corroborated by the correlation between the electoral success of European radical right populists and certain empirical indicators of a crisis (i.e. economic instability, unemployment or political dissatisfaction), the under-theorization of the concept makes this interpretation not entirely reliable (2007: 205). Moreover, as suggested by Rovira Kaltwasser (2012: 186), this link applies better to a 'liberal approach' to populism that conceives populism as a 'pathology', as 'a reaction to the malfunctioning of democratic rule', while it seems less appropriate in other approaches. The relevance of a crisis is thus more nuanced in this strand of literature: a crisis can be a facilitating factor, but it is not necessarily a prerequisite for the rise of populism.

Looking at the literature on crises and the rise of populism in the light of Hay's typology, we acknowledge that most authors refer to different types of specific failures using the term 'crisis' uncritically. The success of populism is often interpreted as being the result of an external crisis (economic, financial, political, migrants, traditional values). The term is thus simply used to depict a conjuncture of disorder, chaos or breakdown. However, these are situations of failure that do not necessarily lead to a crisis of problem-solving rationality. Here, the point does not concern just the terminological question. Populist parties have to be understood in relation to their current political and cultural field (Ostiguy 2017; Weyland 2017). Many commentators on European politics highlight the crisis of representation or democracy as the main factor explaining the emergence and success of populist movements. When applied to populism, Hay's typology is fruitful because it requires crisis situations to be considered as dynamic processes that may have different stages, or facets. In this process, populists can exploit the situation but also actively contribute to the emergence of systemic contradictions, which can lead to an actual crisis. At a critical juncture, populists need their anti-populist counterparts (Stavrakakis et al. 2018).

In this perspective, populists cannot be conceived simply as actors reacting to external crises, but rather as actors that actively perform and spread a sense of crisis. According to Moffitt (2015: 195), it is exactly this performance of crisis that provides populists with 'an effective way to divide "the people" and their other, and to legitimate strong leadership by presenting themselves as voices of the sovereign people'. Populists can, therefore, intervene in those situations that Hay has called *failure*, *catastrophic equilibrium* and *tipping point*, and, through their action, ensure that these contradictions are clearly perceived among citizens and push the system towards the moment of decisive intervention (Table 1).

Table 1 Contradictions, decisive interventions and populist interventions

	Moment of decisive intervention	*Moment of indecisive intervention or non-intervention*
Subjectively perceived contradictions	**CRISIS**	🡐 Catastrophic equilibrium
Unperceived contradictions	🡑 Tipping point	🡔 Failure

➔ = Populist Interventions

Adapted from Hay (1995)

Two components—one real, referred to as systemic failure, and another symbolic, referred to as the public construction of crisis—are thus mobilized by populists and become part of an irreducible dialectic (Stavrakakis et al. 2018). Populists exploit failures, catastrophic equilibria and tipping points through the politicization of the specific issues that underlie them (i.e. unemployment, border control, corruption, Islamic veil, etc.). While politicization—the process through which issues 'are thematised as contingent and controversial topics' (Palonen 2005: 44), becoming subjects of political confrontation among parties and citizens—is a process common to all political actors, populists, bringing every issue into their Manichean vision of society, create a sense of crisis and 'use that sense to inject an urgency and an importance into their message' (Taggart 2004: 275). Populists therefore exploit the contradictions of the system and contribute to amplifying them, in real and symbolic terms, through the politicization of broad or narrow issues related to them. They are performing the crisis (Moffitt 2015) by giving it a discursive reality. As a communication style, populism benefits from the era of polarization and conflict-friendly communication (Blumler 2016; Reinemann et al. 2019)

This is how things normally work when contradictions are endogenous, determined by factors internal to the political system. But when contradictions are exogenous, determined by external shocks, their politicization is more complex, since causal attribution of responsibility is not always possible. This is particularly true for those situations determined by accidental causes or natural disasters such as floods, earthquakes, droughts and hurricanes. Stone (1989: 284) explains that 'these phenomena are devoid of purpose, either in their actions or consequences. In fact, one cannot properly speak of actions here, but only of occurrences. This is the realm of accident and fate'. These accidents are difficult to politicize since they are caused by 'events beyond human control'. They postulate a kind of innocence: no one can exert control over this kind of accident and therefore no one can be blamed. In order to become a political crisis, these kinds of accidents have to be framed as such by agents who have an interest in acting like that. In other words, they need to be politicized.

The COVID-19 health crisis fits perfectly into this kind of framework, where there is a priori no political purpose or direct responsibility for the origin of the pandemic. Such a situation meets the definition of a crisis since both decisive intervention and public awareness of the problem are present. The peculiar nature of this crisis, however, requires further efforts to understand how populists can politicize such an issue and possibly benefit from it. Thus, while governments seek to steer the problem away from the intentional and towards the realm of nature (i.e. managing the COVID-19 crisis as a non-political, science-based task), the other side, which often includes populists, tries to push the problem into the realm of human intention, in order to politicize it.

4 Politicization of the Pandemic Crisis

'Politicization' has long been a key concept in the study of politics. In the European tradition of social and political theory, the term connotes the process through which a given phenomenon or issue enters the sphere of 'the political' and thus turns into a target of contention, a hub for conflicts, a space open to alternatives and controversies (Palonen 2003). In the American tradition of behavioural and empirical political science, the same term tends to signify a narrower dynamic, whereby the visibility of a given phenomenon or issue suddenly increases, attracting public interest and triggering mobilization and 'voice' (Easton 1957; Verba 1960). Additionally, 'de-politicization' has become a classical concept. In the wake of Carl Schmitt's thinking (2008), in the European tradition de-politicization is seen as the removal of a given phenomenon or issue from the realm of 'the political', or a preventative denial of its political character (Rancière 1995; Wood and Flinders 2014). In the American tradition, however, de-politicization mostly indicates a set of narrower processes such as a diminishing interest in politics and participation, the hollowing out of the public sphere, and power exercises aimed at thwarting potential oppositions (Pharr and Putnam 2000; Roberts 2017). On both sides of the Atlantic, de-politicization dynamics have attracted increasing attention—empirically and analytically—in the context of research on technocratic policy-making and anti-politics (Fawcett et al. 2017).

In the last few decades, scholars have mainly used the concept of politicization within three different strands of literature (Zürn 2019). Firstly, at the domestic level, politicization has been mainly studied as a process of de-politicization and re-politicization, especially in investigations of the decline of the class divide, offset by the globalization divide between integrationists and demarcationists (Kriesi et al. 2012) or between cosmopolitans and communitarians (de Wilde et al. 2019; Hooghe and Marks 2017). Secondly, the concept has been widely applied to the process of EU integration and studied through three key dimensions: the salience of the EU and EU related issues, their contentiousness and the expansion of actors engaged with the EU (de Wilde 2011; Statham and Trenz 2012; Hutter and Kriesi 2019). Thirdly, the study of politicization of international institutions has mainly focused on the ongoing transnationalization of social protests (Della Porta 2007; Della Porta and Caiani 2009).

Scholars who have studied politicization in its entirety from the perspective of political theory have found that the term throws up different facets of a complex process and that more clarity is needed, starting with a specific vocabulary (Palonen 2003; Hay 2007).

Alongside this literature, other scholars have dealt with similar processes applied to narrower contexts, such as the emergence of an issue as salient within the political field. Erik Neveu (2015), focusing on the development of public problems, defines it as a multi-stage process through which a private and non-political issue could be transformed into a public problem with a political scope. An issue needs to be constructed, performed and framed as a problem on the public agenda to be perceived as such (Gamson 1990). Entrepreneurs of a public problem—ordinary citizens, stakeholders or political actors—need to implement a series of actions to introduce a specific issue into the political realm (Gusfield 1981). This means framing the issue within the common political divides or conflicts at stake in the political field, or, with more difficulty, pushing the issue as a new divide. Among these actions, the 'naming, blaming, claiming' trilogy (Felstiner et al. 1980) is noteworthy when adapted to public problems (Orsini 2002; Zittoun 2014). 'Naming' refers to the action of defining a private or public situation as unfair and worthy of being politically addressed since it produces individual or collective damage or injuries. 'Blaming' is the action through which one or more social or political actors are identified as responsible for the given problem. Finally, 'claiming' indicates the action of proposing and supporting a solution to the problem (Neveu 2015: 41–94).

In the light of this literature, we propose to combine the process of politicization with the three actions identified by Felstiner et al. (1980) in order to define a framework for the analysis of the *politicization of issues* (Table 2). We argue that an issue, to be politicized, should follow three stages in which distinct processes, actions, objects of contention and outputs follow one another. In the phase of the *emergence* of a problem, the action of 'naming' brings a given issue into the political field and allows political agents to earn a place as legitimate players in the crisis-solving process; in the *confrontation* phase, the attribution of accountability and ownership of the issue is determined through the 'blaming' action; finally, in the *managing* phase, the action of 'claiming' refers to the confrontation of issue-specific solutions.

Table 2 Politicization of public problems/issues

Phase	*Action*	*Contention*	*Output*
Emergence	Naming	Political vs. non-political status of the problem/issue	One or more political or social actors identify a specific problem/issue as a problem/issue with a public scope and political nature The issue becomes a new political divide or opposition
Confrontation	Blaming	Attribution of accountability and ownership of the problem/issue	One or more political or social actors blame other actors for not facing the problem, or not facing it with the necessary urgency and effectiveness
Managing	Claiming	Alternative problem/issue-specific solutions	One or more political or social actors propose a solution and claim the ability to solve the problem/issue

These are also the steps of the political process traditionally followed by populist movements in order to trigger and perform a crisis through which they gain legitimacy: ***naming*** the crisis by identifying failures and elevating the crisis level; ***blaming*** those responsible who acted against the interests of the people, using the media; and finally, ***claiming*** new solutions. This framework will allow us to study the politicization of the COVID-19 issue by looking at the divide between the political and the non-political status of the issue, disputes about different stakes and their relative priority in managing the crisis, and issue-specific and policy-related contentions about COVID-19. The suddenness of the pandemic is interesting, since there is no previous issue ownership at stake.

5 Aims, Framework and Structure of the Book

In the light of the above, the book aims to provide an initial overview of how populist parties reacted during the COVID-19 pandemic crisis. The general research question asks whether populists have benefited from the COVID-19 crisis (RQ1), gaining centrality in the political field and/or using the crisis to push forward new opposition lines. Through a comparative approach, it focuses especially on two sub-questions: How have populists adapted their discourse to the pandemic crisis (RQ1a)? And how have populists politicized the COVID-19 issue (RQ1b)? Besides systemic differences, our assumption is that populists' ability to politicize the COVID-19 issue has been key to their taking advantage of the crisis in terms of relevance in the political debate and citizens' opinion. In addition, since populists have achieved key policy victories and survived the experience of government in recent years (Albertazzi and McDonnell 2015) by maintaining a high level of politization and polarization on controversial issues (Pappas 2019), a second research question asks whether populists in power and populists in opposition have faced COVID-19 in a similar or a different way (RQ2). While the classical divides seem (at least temporarily) to have weakened, we posit that the COVID-19 crisis has opened a window of opportunity for traditional populist claims such as those about controlling borders or against the (pharmaceutical and scientific) elites, with claims tailored for the crisis, such as the limitation of public freedoms or support for new conspiracy theories.

The analysis aims to identify the main features of populist action by focusing on the leaders' statements and their political initiatives over a period of four months, from January to May. This period covers three different phases: (a) pre-COVID phase, when the COVID-19 crisis was elsewhere, and there were no contagions or national outbreaks; (b) the phase of virus spread and containment measures, when COVID-19 was widely diffuse in the country and restrictive measures were taken by the political authorities; and (c) the mitigation of contagion phase, when the virus spread was under control in the country and restrictive measures were eased or removed. With regard to official activities on their websites and social media profiles, two distinct analyses were run. On the one hand, the key elements of populism—the people, the elites, and out-groups—were analysed in order to understand how they discourses unfolded in this crisis situation and whether they changed compared to a routine period (RQ1a). On the other hand, an assessment was made of how populists defined and attempted to politicize the COVID-19 issue, using the framework of politicization based on the *naming*, *blaming*, *claiming* formula (Table 2).

The variety of cases analysed (hard hit by the crisis or otherwise) and types of populism (right-wing, left-wing, in power or not) allow this book to contribute to the literature on crises and populism, to account for similarities and differences and to define patterns among different types of

Table 3 Impact of COVID-19 in the cases selected (10 June 2020)

	Reported deaths	*Reported deaths per 100,000 population*	*Impact of COVID-19*
Spain	27,136	58.1	High
UK	40,883	61.5	
Italy	34,043	56.3	
France	29,296	43.7	
Germany	8729	10.5	Medium
Hungary	550	5.6	
Poland	1183	3.1	Low
Czech Republic	328	3.1	

Source European Centre for Disease Prevention and Control (www.ecdc.europa.eu/en/cases-2019-ncov-eueea)

populism (RQ2). We gathered data from eight European countries from various geographical regions of the European Union that were differently affected by the pandemic (Table 3). Four countries were in a critical situation: Spain, Italy, France and the United Kingdom. Conversely, two countries were affected very little by the pandemic (Poland and Czech Republic). Finally, we add two countries experiencing a medium situation (Germany and Hungary). These eight countries implemented and experimented with different policies to face the crisis. We also mixed different political situations (Table 4): countries with governing populist parties (Italy, Hungary, Poland, Czech Republic and Spain) with ones with non-governing populist parties (France, Germany, UK).

Table 4 Populists parties in the cases selected

	Impact of COVID-19		
Relevance of populism	*High*	*Medium*	*Low*
In power	Italy (M5S) Spain (Podemos)	Hungary (Fidesz and KDNP)	Poland (PiS) Czech Republic (ANO)
In opposition	Italy (League) UK (Brexit Party) France (RN and LFI) Spain (Vox)	Germany (AfD)	Czech Republic (SPD and KSČM) Poland (Konfederacja)

References

Aalberg, T., Esser, F., C. Reinemann, C., Strömbäck, J., de Vreese, C. (Eds.). (2017). *Populist Political Communication in Europe*. New York: Routledge.

Albertazzi, D., & McDonnell, D. (2015). *Populists in Power*. Abingdon, Oxon and New York: Routledge.

Arditi, B. (2007). *Politics on the Edges of Liberalism: Difference, Populism, Revolution, Agitation*. Edinburgh: Edinburgh University Press.

Betz, H. G., & Johnson, C. (2004). Against the Current—Stemming the Tide: The Nostalgic Ideology of the Contemporary Radical Populist Right. *Journal of Political Ideologies, 9*(3), 311–327.

Blumler, J. (2016). The Fourth Age of Political Communication. *Politiques de Communication, 6*(1), 19–30.

Brubaker, R. (2017). Why Populism? *Theory and Society, 46*, 357–385.

Canovan, M. (1999). Trust the People! *Populism and the Two Faces of Democracy, Political Studies, 47*(1), 2–16.

Conti, N. (2018). National Political Elites, the EU, and the Populist Challenge. *Politics, 38*(3), 361–377.

de Vreese, C. H., Esser, F., Aalberg, T., Reinemann, C., & Stanyer, J. (2018). Populism as an Expression of Political Communication Content and Style: A New Perspective. *The International Journal of Press/Politics, 23*(4), 423–438.

de Wilde, P. (2011). No Polity for Old Politics? A Framework for Analyzing the Politicization of European Integration. *Journal of European Integration, 33*(5), 559–575.

De Wilde, P., Koopmans, R., Merkel, W., Strijbis, O., & Zürn, M. (Eds.). (2019). *The Struggle Over Borders: Cosmopolitanism and Communitarianism*. Cambridge: Cambridge University Press.

Della Porta, D. (Ed.). (2007). *The Global Justice Movement: Cross-National and Transnational Perspectives*. Boulder: Paradigm.

Della Porta, D., & Caiani, M. (2009). *Social Movements and Europeanization*. Oxford: Oxford University Press.

Easton, D. (1957). An Approach to the Analysis of Political Systems. *World Politics, 9*(3), 383–400.

Fawcett, P., Flinders, M., Wood, M., & Hay, C. (Eds.). (2017). *Anti-politics, Depoliticization, and Governance*. Oxford: Oxford University Press.

Felstiner, W. L. F., Abel, R. L., & Sarat, A. (1980). The Emergence and Transformation of Disputes: Naming, Blaming, Claiming… *Law & Society Review, 15*(3/4): 631–654.

Gamson, W. (1990). *The Strategy of Social Protest*. Belmont: Wadsworth Pub.

Gramsci, A. (1971). *Selections From Prison Notebooks*. London: Lawrence & Wishart.

Gusfield, J. (1981). *The Culture of Public Problems: Drinking-Driving and the Symbolic Order*. Chicago: University of Chicago Press.

Habermas, J. (1975). *Legitimation Crisis*. Boston: Beacon Press.
Hay, C. (1995). Narratives of the New Right and Constructions of Crisis. *Rethinking Marxism, 8*(2), 60–76.
Hay, C. (1999). Crisis and the Structural Transformation of the State: Interrogating the Process of Change. *British Journal of Politics and International Relations, 1*(2), 317–344.
Hay, C. (2007). *Why We Hate Politics*. Cambridge: Polity Press.
Hooghe, L., & Marks, G. (2017). Cleavage Theory Meets Europe's Crises: Lipset, Rokkan, and the Transnational Cleavage. *Journal of European Public Policy, 25*(1), 109–135.
Hutter, S., & Kriesi, H. (2019). Politicizing Europe in Times of Crisis. *Journal of European Public Policy, 26*(7), 996–1017.
Jagers, J., & Walgrave, S. (2007). Populism as Political Communication Style: An Empirical Study of Political Parties' Discourse in Belgium. *European Journal of Political Research, 46*(3), 319–345.
Kneuer, M. (2019). The Tandem of Populism and Euroscepticism: A Comparative Perspective in the Light of the European Crises. *Contemporary Social Science, 14*(1), 26–42.
Knight, A. (1998). Populism and Neo-Populism in Latin America, Especially Mexico. *Journal of Latin American Studies, 30*(2), 223–248.
Koselleck, R. (2006). Crisis. *Journal of the History of Ideas, 67*(2), 357–400.
Kriesi, H. (2015) Populism. Concepts and Conditions for Its Rise in Europe. *Comunicazione politica, 16*(2), 175–193.
Kriesi, H., & Pappas, T. (Eds.). (2015). *European Populism in the Shadow of the Great Recession*. Colchester: ECPR Press.
Kriesi, H., Grande, E., Dolezal, M., Helbling, M., Hutter, S., Höglinger, D., et al. (2012). *Political conflict in Western Europe*. Cambridge: Cambridge University Press.
Kriesi, H., Grande, E., Lachat, R., Dolezal, M., Bornschier, S., Frey & T. (2006). Globalization and the Transformation of the National Political Space: Six European Countries Compared. *European Journal of Political Research, 45*(6), 921–957.
Laclau, E. (1977). *Politics and Ideology in Marxist Theory*. London: New Left Books.
Laclau, E. (2005). *On Populist Reason*. London: Verso.
Mair, P. (2002). Populist Democracy vs Party Democracy. In Y. Mény & Y. Surel (Eds.), *Democracies and the Populist Challenge*. London: Palgrave Macmillan.
Marx, K. (1981). *Capital Volume III* (D. Fernbach, Trans.) London: Penguin Books.
Moffitt, B. (2015). How to Perform Crisis: A Model for Understanding the Key Role of Crisis in Contemporary Populism. *Government and Opposition, 50*(2), 189–217.

Moffitt, B. (2016). *The Global Rise of Populism: Performance, Political Style, Representation*. Stanford: Stanford University Press.
Mouffe C. (2005). *On the Political*. Abingdon and New York: Routledge.
Mudde, C. (2004). The Populist Zeitgeist. *Government & Opposition, 39*(4), 541–563.
Mudde, C. (2007). *Populist Radical Right Parties in Europe*. Cambridge: Cambridge University Press.
Mudde, C., & Rovira Kaltwasser, C. (2017). *Populism: A Very Short Introduction*. Oxford and New York: Oxford University Press.
Müller, J. W. (2016). *What Is populism?*. Philapelphia: University of Pennsylvania Press.
Neveu, E. (2015). *Sociologie des problèmes publics*. Paris: Armand Colin.
Orsini, M. (2002). The Politics of Naming, Blaming and Claiming: HIV, Hepatitis C and the Emergence of Blood Activism in Canada. *Canadian Journal of Political Science / Revue Canadienne de Science Politique, 35*(3), 475–498.
Ostiguy, P. (2017). Populism: A Socio-Cultural Approach. In C. Rovira Kaltwasser, P. Taggart, P. Ochoa Espejo, & P. Ostiguy (Eds.), *The Oxford Handbook of Populism* (pp. 73–97). Oxford: Oxford University Press.
Palonen, K. (2003). Four Times of Politics: Policy, Polity, Politicking, and Politicization. *Alternatives, 28*(2), 171–186.
Palonen, K. (2005). The Politics of Conceptual History. *Contributions to the History of Concepts, 1*(1), 37–50.
Pappas, T. S. (2019). Populists in Power. *Journal of Democracy, 30*(2), 70–84.
Pharr, S. J., & Putnam, R. D. (Eds.). (2000). *Disaffected Democracies: What's Troubling the Trilateral Countries?*. Princeton: Princeton University Press.
Rancière, J. (1995). *On the Shores of Politics*. London: Verso.
Reinemann, C., Stanyer, J., Aalberg, T., Esser, F., & de Vreese, C. (Eds.). (2019). *Communicating Populism: Comparing Interactions Between Politicians, Media, and Citizens Across Europe*. New York: Routledge.
Roberts, A. (2017). *Four Crises of American democracy: Representation, Mastery, Discipline, Anticipation*. Oxford: Oxford University Press.
Roberts, K. (1995). Neoliberalism and the Transformation of Populism in Latin America: The Peruvian Case. *World Politics, 48*(1), 82–116.
Roberts, K. (2015). Populism, Political Mobilizations, and Crises of Political Representation. In C. de la Torre (Ed.), *The Promise and Perils of Populism* (pp. 140–158). Lexington: The University Press of Kentucky.
Rovira Kaltwasser, C. (2012). The Ambivalence of Populism: Threat and Corrective for Democracy. *Democratization, 19*(2), 184–208.
Schmitt, C. (2008). *The Concept of the Political* (Expanded ed.). Chicago: University of Chicago Press.

Statham, P., & Trenz, H. J. (2012). *The Politicization of Europe: Contesting the Constitution in the Mass Media*. London: Routledge.

Stavrakakis, Y., Katsambekis, G., Kioupkiolis, A., Nikisianis, N., & Siomos, T. (2018). Populism, Anti-Populism and Crisis. *Contemporary Political Theory, 17*, 4–27.

Stojarová, V. (2018). Populist, Radical and Extremist Political Parties in Visegrad Countries Vis à Vis the Migration Crisis. In the name of the people and the nation in Central Europe, *Open Political Science, 1*(1), 32–45.

Stone, D. (1989). Causal Stories and the Formation of Policy Agendas. *Political Science Quarterly, 104*(2), 281–300.

Taggart, P. (2004). Populism and Representative Politics in Contemporary Europe. *Journal of Political Ideologies, 9*(3), 269–288.

Taggart, P. (2000). *Populism: Concepts in the Social Sciences*. Buckingham: Open University Press.

Trenz, H.-J., Ruzza, C., & Guiraudon, V. (Eds.). (2015). *Europe's Prolonged Crisis: The Making or the Unmaking of a Political Union*. London: Palgrave.

Urbinati, N. (2019). Political Theory of Populism. *Annual Review of Political Science, 22*, 111–127.

Verba, S. (1960). Political Behavior and Politics. *World Politics, 12*(2), 280–291.

Weyland, K. (1999). Neoliberal Populism in Latin America and Eastern Europe. *Comparative Politics, 31*(4), 379–401.

Weyland, K. (2001). Clarifying a Contested Concept: 'Populism' in the Study of Latin American Politics. *Comparative Politics, 34*(1), 1–22.

Weyland, K. (2017). Populism: A Political-Strategic Approach. In C. Rovira Kaltwasser, P. Taggart, P. Ochoa Espejo, & P. Ostiguy (Eds.), *The Oxford Handbook of Populism* (pp. 48–72). Oxford: Oxford University Press.

Wood, M., & Flinders, M. (2014). Rethinking Depoliticisation: Beyond the Governmental. *Policy & Politics, 42*(2), 151–170.

Zittoun, P. (2014). Creating Social Disorder: Constructing, Propagating and Policitising Social Problems. In *The Political Process of Policymaking: Studies in the Political Economy of Public Policy*. London: Palgrave Macmillan.

Zürn, M. (2019). Politicization Compared: At National, European, and Global Levels. *Journal of European Public Policy, 26*(7), 977–995.

CHAPTER 2

UK: Between Managed Moderation and Far-Right Conspiracy Theories

Osman Sahin and *Bogdan Ianosev*

1 Introduction

The outbreak of the pandemic in the UK was perceived to be inevitable as other European countries, most notably Italy, had already succumbed to COVID-19. The Johnson government explained that the United Kingdom (UK) was two weeks behind Italy and the NHS could be overwhelmed by COVID-19 very much like the Italian health system had been. By mid-March 2020, it became clear in the UK that the pandemic was no longer a 'Chinese problem'. Nevertheless, the UK government seemed from the beginning insufficiently prepared. The government was slow in stopping international flights from regions with high infection rates, which probably contributed to the spread of COVID-19. Early in the pandemic, there was a shortage in personal protective equipment, causing hundreds of the NHS staff to be infected with the virus. These factors provided a fertile ground for populist politics. Despite this fact, Farage and his Brexit Party kept a rather low profile during the pandemic.

O. Sahin (✉) · B. Ianosev
Glasgow Caledonian University, Glasgow, Scotland, UK

G. Bobba and N. Hubé (eds.), *Populism and the Politicization of the COVID-19 Crisis in Europe*,
https://doi.org/10.1007/978-3-030-66011-6_2

This was due to two reasons. First, populism in the UK is mostly geared towards Brexit. Therefore, the pandemic at least at the beginning was not on Farage's radar. Second, UK populists' influence on public opinion is mostly limited to Brexit. This does not mean that Farage abstained from politicizing the issue and using it to advance his agenda.

2 Political Context

The British variant of the latest wave of populism engulfing the world in the past few decades can be traced back to the United Kingdom Independence Party (UKIP). UKIP was founded in 1993 by members of the Anti-Federalist League. At the beginning, UKIP was considered a splinter group of the Conservative Party and was originally designed as a single-issue, policy-seeking party having the sole aim of facilitating the UK's exit from the European Union (EU) (Ford and Goodwin 2014; Rekawek 2015). Since its early days, UKIP sought to pressure the Conservative Party into adopting a harsher stance on Europe, opposed plans for further European integration and sought the withdrawal of the UK from the EU (Ford and Goodwin 2014). UKIP followed into the footsteps of an established British political tradition of Euroscepticism (Bale 2018). Although some scholars argue that the marriage between Euroscepticism and populism was present from the first stages of UKIP's historical development (Tournier-Sol 2015), others suggest that populism was rather a subsequent, although invaluable addition to the party's repertoire (Taggart 2017; Bale 2018).

By 2010, UKIP switched to being a vote-seeking party mainly due to the contribution of then-party leader Nigel Farage who popularized UKIP's single issue by connecting it to populist backlash towards current immigration policies. This afforded UKIP to set the limelight on the long-standing issue the party was promoting ever since its inception, and which never before truly captured the full attention of the British electorate (Ford and Goodwin 2014; Tournier-Sol 2015; Bale 2018). Banking on voters' understanding that leaving the EU would increase the possibility of restricting immigration, UKIP, as the only party openly advocating exit from the EU, could therefore credibly signal that they mean business (Rekawek 2015; Bale 2018). Nigel Farage's appeal to voters was straightforwardly right-wing populist, anti-establishment, nativist, neo-nostalgic, and neo-traditionalist (Ford and Goodwin 2014; Reed 2016; Breeze 2019).

For most of its existence so far, UKIP never really took off in the polls. The party started off with a meagre 1% of the vote in 1994 European Parliament (EP) election, while settling for a mere 0.3% of the vote in the 1997 general election. It was only after 2010 that UKIP experienced a surge in popularity, which culminated with the 2014 EP election, when UKIP won the first place in the popular vote by securing 27.5% of the votes (Ford and Goodwin 2014). In the 2014 by-election, support for main parties (Labour, Liberal Democrats, and Conservatives) plummeted, while support for UKIP rose by 36% (Ford and Goodwin 2014; Tournier-Sol 2015). Ultimately, the biggest contribution of UKIP was in succeeding to pressure the Conservatives into holding an EU membership referendum (Rekawek 2015; Taggart 2017). The referendum was held on June 23, 2016, and Britain voted to leave the EU by a close margin, leading to a deeply polarized political environment ever since. After the referendum, support for UKIP practically collapsed. By then, however, Nigel Farage had already left UKIP, and, followed by several UKIP MEPs, in January 2019, formed the Brexit Party, which later that year ended up winning the 2019 EP election with 31.6% of the vote and 29 seats.

Nigel Farage's Brexit Party has clung onto the 2016 Leave campaign promises in its fight to see through Britain's exit from the EU, as Brexit negotiations are set to be concluded by the end of 2020. Although largely debunked, Leave campaign slogans seem today as valid as ever, judging by Farage's electoral success in EP elections, and by the overwhelming victory of Prime Minister (PM) Boris Johnson's Conservative Party in the 2019 general election, after campaigning on the very same messaging (Tormey 2020). The election result seemed a logical outcome of all the 'good' work done by the Leave campaign in 2016, of which Johnson was an integral part. The campaign used simple stories and false but intuitive narratives while depicting migrants and politicians alike in populist Manichean terms of outgroups competing for British resources. Similarly, the EU was portrayed as an imperialist superpower planning to subdue Britain. To all this, Brexit was supposed to be the answer, the magical one-shot win-all option, aptly summarized by PM Boris Johnson's 2019 electoral motto 'Get Brexit Done'. In this way, populism and Brexit came together and decided the election results. Finally, in July 2020, UKIP polled at about 2%, while the Brexit Party had garnered only 1% of popular support, once Brexit was finally being done (Table 1).

Table 1 Main UK political parties (>5% in the last European election. Because first-past-the-post system is used in general elections, the threshold for the UK case is calculated considering the European elections instead of the general elections)

Political party	*2019 general election*		*2019 European election*	
	Vote shares (%)	*Seats*	*Vote shares (%)*	*Seats*
In power				
The Conservative and Unionist Party	43.6	365	9.1	4
In opposition				
The Labour Party	32.2	203	14.1	10
Brexit Party	2	0	30.5	29
Greens	2.7	1	4	7
Liberal Democrats	11.5	11	19.6	16

3 COVID-19 Diffusion and Political Measures

In the UK, during the *first phase* of the pandemic, the attention of the public and the media was focused on Italy, which was the first epicentre of the pandemic in Europe. This was despite the fact that the first COVID-19 diagnosis in the UK was recorded as early as 31 January. Accordingly, one can argue that the initial reaction of the public and the state authorities to the COVID-19 pandemic was rather weak. No quarantine or extra safety checks were introduced for international passengers arriving from Southeast Asia or Europe. As of March 18, the UK still did not impose a ban on non-essential travel whereas the EU banned all non-essential travel from outside the European Union.[1] The only noticeable action of the government was to advise its citizens to abstain from any non-essential travel for the next 30 days. It also advised its citizens abroad to return to the country if they can. Despite the pressure from the opposition, Boris Johnson declined to treat the situation as an emergency, which was also apparent in his unwillingness to hold a so-called Cobra meeting—namely meetings with Prime Minister advisers in times of national emergencies—even after the pandemic started to spread throughout Europe in late February.

[1] PWC, COVID-19: Global travel restrictions, entry bans and quarantine measures, 18 March 2020.

The *second phase* started in March where local cases with no travel history started to spike. As of March 10, 2020, the number of tests reached 26,000 with 373 people testing positive. Six people died because of COVID-19 by March 10. Only 18 days later, the government reported 17,089 positive cases while the death toll reached 1019 people. These figures included PM Johnson who tested positive on March 27, and who was hospitalized due to breathing difficulties. This new reality check compelled the government to reconsider its strategy. While the government previously insisted that based on scientific advice, a 'herd immunity' approach was the best strategy to deal with the pandemic, they had to backtrack from this position after heavy criticism and after an influential report from the Imperial College London. This report predicted that, if left unchecked, the government strategy would cause as much as 260,000 deaths and the NHS would most likely 'break' under the increasing number of patients. Hence, the government had to announce a lockdown on March 23, 2020. Johnson announced that all non-essential shops must close effective immediately and people must stay at home. He also advised the people not to go to shopping except for essentials such as food and medicine. Despite these measures, the Johnson government was criticized for acting late as London had already buckled under the weight of the pandemic. Throughout April 2020, cases in the UK increased so much so that by the end of May 2020 it was clear that the UK was one of the worst performing countries in fighting the pandemic. The death toll in the UK passed 50,000 on June 2, making it the highest in Europe (Fig 1 and Table 2).

The UK started to flatten the curve towards the beginning of May, which enabled the government to introduce some relaxation measures to the lockdown. Thus, the *third phase* started on May 13, 2020. Johnson encouraged people in England to go back to work if they cannot work from home. He also advised citizens to avoid public transport when possible. Other devolved nations, Scotland, Wales and Northern Ireland, however, did not rush to follow Johnson's footsteps as their governments argued that it was still too early to introduce a relaxation of lockdown measures. This also signified the beginning of diverging approaches the devolved nations took during the third phase. Especially Scotland's First Minister Nicola Sturgeon was quite cautious to follow the 10 Downing Street as she argued that England was too hasty to open up the economy. Nevertheless, the situation has almost normalized all across the UK especially in July. Foreign flights to major hubs have resumed with important

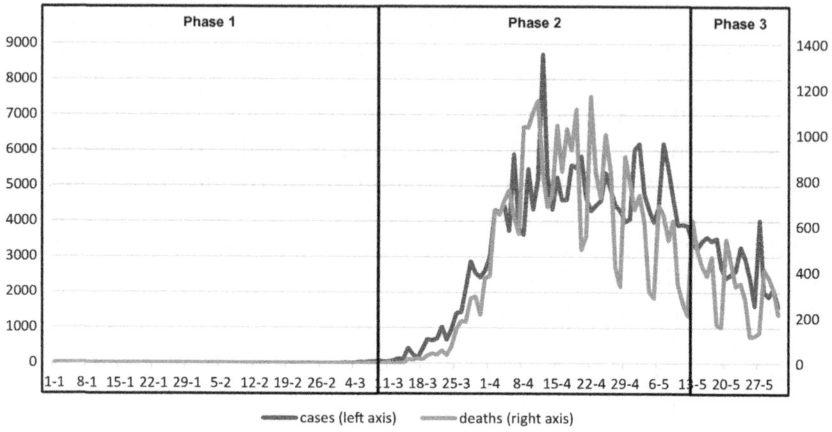

Fig. 1 Daily death toll and new cases in UK (*Source* European Centre for Disease Prevention and Control. Phase 1: pre-COVID-19; Phase 2: spread and containment measures; Phase 3: contagion mitigation)

Table 2 COVID-19 pandemic in UK

Cases	289,140
Total deaths	40,883
Total recovered	N/A
Cases for 1 M pop	4260
Deaths for 1 M pop	602

Source www.worldometers.info/coronavirus/ (update 10/6/2020)

exceptions such as the United States. Pubs, restaurants and hairdressers were allowed to open throughout the UK in July while schools resumed their normal curriculum in August 2020.

4 Populist Discourse at the Time of COVID-19

Nigel Farage took the opportunity of the pandemic to fight for some questionable goals while deploying established right-wing populist tropes. The thematical proximity of right-wing populism to conspiracism as established in previous research (Bergmann 2018) is also evident in the communication of Farage on social media and in his political messaging in the media and at rallies. Given that Nigel Farage had left his seat in the European Parliament (EP) as a result of Brexit before the pandemic captured the national awareness in Britain, most of his statements on COVID-19 have been uttered either in the media or posted on social media.

Nigel Farage adapted his discourse to the COVID-19 crisis mainly in two ways. First, and probably least problematic, Farage criticized the latency with which the British government introduced measures to counteract the spread of the pandemic. He also criticized the government for providing the inadequate response of adopting a 'herd immunity' approach. To this end, he pointed out that PM Boris Johnson's policy of herd immunity would likely lead to 400,000 thousand deaths, from his own estimates, or alternatively to 260,000 deaths, citing an estimate by the Imperial College London.[2] Second, his central position on the pandemic was twofold: (1) he argued against the lockdown and against what he believed were harsh enforcement measures, likening the UK government to East Germany (Farage's Facebook page, 30/03/2020) while at the same time (2) decrying the government's decision to both allow inbound flights during lockdown and the 'daily import of spreaders' from high-risk countries such as China, Italy, or the United States (US) (Farage's Facebook page, 02/04/2020). Within his central position on the pandemic, he vilified China as the paradigmatic enemy of 'the West' and attempted to promote outrage over the silent 'invasion' of migrants on the beaches of England (Farage's Facebook page, 20/05/2020).

Farage echoed Trump in blaming China for the pandemic, claiming that the Chinese government caused COVID-19. He also called for a tougher stance on China.[3] For Farage, China was 'a surveillance state that infected the world with a deadly disease' (Farage's Facebook page, 20/04/2020) that expels American journalists and oppresses religious minorities, that caused three viruses (i.e., SARS, the swine flu, and COVID-19), and that initially suppressed the truth about COVID-19 costing thousands of lives worldwide. China is also held responsible for global pollution and was ultimately characterized by Farage as '*this*

[2] Farage, N., The Virus Is Yet Another Reason to Rethink the West's Relationship With China. *Newsweek*, 18 March 2020.

[3] Harris, K, Nigel Farage Lashes Out at China over Coronavirus: 'We Need to Get TOUGH!'. *Express*, 2 June 2020.

murderous atrocity that has brought the world such misery'.[4] He then assumed a novel role for his Brexit Party: to hold China to account.[5]

During the pandemic, in an article peroration published in *Newsweek.co.uk*, Nigel Farage deployed most of the tropes associated with white supremacist conspiracy theories. These included: 'the West' (framed as a unified and distinct body in opposition to China); 'the Left' (an amorphous pseudo-entity embodying all which does not conform to the right-wing populist notion of 'the [in this case mainly white] people') collaborating with proponents of 'political correctness'; environmental movements such as 'extinction rebellion' (the youth movement that has supposedly 'brought British cities to a standstill') or the (imagined) 'Green Lobby' who are seen to inflict 'chaos on our society'; and even the World Health Organization (WHO) is depicted as being pro-China. Farage ends his peroration by calling for an all-out boycott on Chinese products, as well as calling for PM Johnson to deny Chinese company Huawei the right to build Britain's 5G network (Farage's Facebook page, 20/04/2020). He also claimed that the British establishment had previously sold Britain out to EU leaders in Brussels and is now selling Britain out to Beijing (Farage's Facebook page, 19/04/2020).

Farage's populist anti-'Left' discourse mirrored US president Trump's attempt to pinpoint yet another term for the collectively conspiring enemy: 'far-left fascism'. To this end, Farage referred to the government's stay-at-home advice as 'house arrest' (Farage's Facebook page, 30/03/2020). Farage portrayed 'the Left' and all its subsidiaries as conspiring to destroy the British way of life and to strip citizens' rights and freedoms, as 'the Left' is beholden to Chinese interests and would not criticize the Chinese government in fear of losing lucrative business deals and that the political 'establishment' has been 'payed off by China' (Farage's Facebook page, 22/02/2020). 'The Green Lobby' was depicted as a malevolent agent to which Farage ascribed intentionality and emotion (e.g., 'happy to inflict chaos').[6] He implicitly referred to alt-right conspiracy theories by mentioning 'globalists' in relation to 'the Left'

[4] Farage, N., The Virus Is Yet Another Reason to Rethink the West's Relationship With China. *Newsweek*, 18 March 2020.

[5] Harris, K, Nigel Farage Lashes Out at China over Coronavirus: We Need to Get TOUGH!'. *Express*, 2 June 2020.

[6] Farage, N., The Virus Is Yet Another Reason to Rethink the West's Relationship With China. *Newsweek*, 18 March 2020.

and to the establishment as promoting globalization against the will of the people (Farage's Facebook page, 01/05/2020). Farage also blamed globalization for the pandemic partly because globalization allegedly leads powerful figures to play in the hands of the Chinese government.[7]

Finally, during the COVID-19 pandemic, Farage engaged in fearmongering over a small number of migrants crossing the English Channel illegally. He breached government lockdown advice to travel 100 miles to East Sussex to document the alleged migrant 'invasion'.[8] After being reprimanded by the police for breaching social distancing rules, Farage called the police visit 'lunacy'.[9] He further suggested that migrants are carrying COVID-19 (reminiscent of established dehumanization strategies deployed by right-wing populists against migrants and refugees), and claimed that the media is silent about the 'invasion' (Farage's Facebook page, 26/04/2020). He further claimed that French ships were 'escorting' migrant boats into British waters and tried to 'cover it up' (Farage's Facebook page, 27/05/2020). He also called for a stop on flights bringing seasonal workers from Romania into western Europe as he suggested that seasonal workers might spread the virus in Britain (Farage's Facebook page, 18/04/2020).

5 The Politicization of COVID-19 Issue by Populists

During the pandemic, the Johnson government avoided using a discourse that could have contributed to the politicization of the crisis. Instead, on several occasions, Johnson emphasized that the government would be guided by scientific advice. Indeed, early in the pandemic, the Chief Scientific Advisor Patrick Vallance became a household name as PM Johnson included him in the daily COVID-19 press conferences where Vallance explained the government strategy to fight the pandemic. When the herd immunity approach, initially cherished by the UK government, drew heavy criticism by the public health authorities (i.e. the Imperial College London report), the government overrode its initial decision and imposed

[7] Ibid.

[8] Nigel Farage, *Talk Radio Interview*, 30 April 2020.

[9] 'Lunacy', Says Nigel Farage After Police Visit over Lockdown Trip. *Politico*, 5 May 2020.

a lockdown throughout the nation. Furthermore, unlike Nigel Farage or the Trump administration, the Johnson government was hesitant to put any blame on China. When conspiracy theories emerged that 5G is behind the spread of COVID-19, the Cabinet Secretary Michael Gove was quick to define these theories as 'dangerous nonsense'.[10]

Unlike the government, however, Nigel Farage chose to politicize the COVID-19 crisis early in the *emergence phase*. On January 23, Farage slammed the Johnson government for its lax response to the outbreak in relation to China.[11] He suggested that all passengers coming from China should have their temperatures checked in the airports. Farage also differed from the government approach in terms of his take on the pandemic. While the government undermined the seriousness of the crisis mostly because of economic concerns, Farage opportunistically used the COVID-19 crisis to suggest a scale down to the UK's relations with the EU and China. For instance, he argued that while the government could monitor flights from China landing back in the UK, it was not possible to monitor those flights landing from China in the rest of Europe. He therefore suggested that the EU freedom of movement did make the UK more vulnerable to the pandemic.[12]

There is a certain overlap between the first phase (*emergence phase*) and the second phase (*confrontation phase*) as Farage moved onto the identification of actors who were responsible for the COVID-19 crisis in the UK. Farage suggested that those who were responsible for the UK's crisis were China, the Johnson government, and migrants. Farage was in the same boat with Donald Trump in blaming China for the pandemic. He argued that before the pandemic, China was a surveillance state; now, it is a surveillance state that infected the world with a deadly disease (Farage's Facebook page, 20/04/2020). In several statements and social media posts during April and May 2020, Farage accused China for the pandemic and asserted that China should let independent investigators into the country to reveal the true scope of its guilt during the spread of the virus. Farage also referred to China several times in his accusations levelled

[10] Gove Warns 5G-Coronavirus Conspiracy Theory Is 'Dangerous Nonsense'. *The Guardian*, 4 April 2020.

[11] Nigel Farage 'Astonished' at UK Government's Response to Coronavirus 'Just a Leaflet?!'. *Daily Express*, 23 January 2020..

[12] Is the EU Holding Up Britain's Coronavirus Response?. *Daily Mail*, 5 February 2020.

against the Johnson government and the establishment. He blamed the Johnson government for being soft on China despite China's share in the pandemic. He suggested the government should learn from the Trump administration. After Trump's announcement that the US is withdrawing its financial support from what Farage defined as the 'pro-China' WHO, he argued that the Johnson government should be ashamed of continuing to fund the WHO (Farage's Facebook page, 14/04/2020). In fact, during the pandemic, Farage emerged as a vocal proponent of the US position on China's role in the pandemic. Farage said that Trump was correct to define COVID-19 as the 'Chinese virus' because, he claimed, China was responsible for the outbreak.[13]

A second target for Farage during the confrontation phase was the Johnson government. Along with his accusations against the government for being subordinated to China, Farage blamed the Johnson government for being incompetent and indecisive in the face of the COVID-19 crisis. After Johnson's announcement in early March 2020 that no immediate steps would be taken against COVID-19, Farage stated that Johnson is failing to show leadership (Farage's Facebook page, 12/03/2020). Furthermore, on several occasions, Farage criticized the government over its lockdown decision, which was announced by PM Johnson on March 23, 2020. He likened the lockdown to a house arrest or home detention.[14] Farage argued that while other measures such as wearing mask or keeping social distance were acceptable, the government decision to impose a total lockdown was going too far as a measure in the fight against the virus.

Another target of Farage during the COVID-19 crisis was irregular and regular migrants. He claimed that COVID-19 diverted attention from what he perceived to be a serious problem. Farage suggested that during the pandemic there had been a 'continuing flow of illegal migrants that makes many of us very angry' (Farage's Facebook page, 24/04/2020). According to Farage, the media was ignoring the flow of these immigrants crossing the English Channel, which he described as 'the beginning of an invasion' (Farage's Facebook page, 08/05/2020). Farage presented

[13] Nigel Farage Facing Backlash After Blaming China for Coronavirus Pandemic. *The National*, 19 March 2020.

[14] Farage, N., Of Course We Must Stop Coronavirus, But Not at the Cost of Becoming a Police State. *The Telegraph*, 30 March 2020.

these immigrants as potential COVID-19 spreaders by arguing that irregular migrants would be neither sent back nor quarantined. Farage also suggested that seasonal workers from abroad (generally from Romania or Poland) who come to the UK to pick fruit or vegetables must be stopped because they are potential spreaders of the virus. In addition, he argued, as many British workers were either out of their jobs or furloughed due to the COVID-19 crisis, they could easily replace the seasonal workers from abroad.

In the following *managing phase*, which started in mid-May, Farage proposed several solutions to deal with the pandemic while criticizing the government for some of its policies. Unlike other populist leaders such as Trump or Bolsonaro, Farage did not despise face masks. On the contrary, he criticized the Johnson government for failing to enforce wearing face masks in the public. Farage argued that anything that could help ease the lockdown (i.e. face masks) should be encouraged (Farage's Facebook page, 16/04/2020). Farage also proposed to stop international flights to the UK whereas the government was reluctant to do so. Despite these proposals, it would be an exaggeration to claim that Nigel Farage had a comprehensive programme to fight the COVID-19 crisis. Instead, his proposals were mostly ad hoc and mostly aiming to curb the severity of the lockdown in the UK. Rather, he benefited from the pandemic to frame China as the new enemy of 'the West' renewing the relevance of his Brexit Party in current affairs.

As for PM Boris Johnson, aside from benefitting from the pronounced populist undertones of the pro-Brexit campaign, and from decades of right-wing, pro-Brexit mainstream media (Cromby 2019), any populist elements inside his discourse surrounding the pandemic were considerably toned down, arguably even non-existent. The mainstream media was also careful to avoid a populist tone in criticizing the Prime Minister. Most of the criticisms towards the government was built upon the premise that the government paid too much attention to the economic implications of measures against the pandemic while overlooking scientific advice. In fact, the media's insistence on publicizing the now-famous Imperial College London report on COVID-19, which argued that herd immunity could cause as much as 260,000 deaths, was probably a major factor in the government's decision to ditch this strategy and impose a total lockdown.

6 Conclusion

Nigel Farage used the pandemic to advance his goal of realizing a no-deal Brexit. Even as polls place the Brexit Party below 2%, his contribution was only ever reflected within the Brexit process. This explains the observed discrepancy between the infinitesimal polling of the Brexit Party on the one hand, and its crushing victory in the 2019 EP election on the other. The relevance of Nigel Farage and his party increases as he is careful to include common right-wing conspiracist tropes in his discourse and as he appears willing to wage a pseudo-crusade against alleged external and internal enemies of Britain and 'the West', such as China and the 'politically correct Left'. This is why Farage chose to employ similar tactics during the pandemic.

Recent electoral success of the British Conservatives suggests that a majority of British voters are still willing to buy what Farage and his more soft-spoken populist counterpart, PM Boris Johnson, are selling. As Britain is rapidly heading towards a no-deal Brexit scenario due to the UK government's apparent unwillingness to strike any kind of deal with the EU, thus fulfilling Farage's long time aim, Farage is careful to confer novel relevancy to his party by setting the new goal of antagonizing China. To this end, Farage added the pandemic to his case against China. At the same time, his opposition to lockdown measures is not so much opposition directed at government policy as it is intended to work as a dog whistle against globalization and the 'oppressive' 'Left' collaborating with and never criticizing China.

References

Bale, T. (2018). Who Leads and Who Follows? The Symbiotic Relationship Between UKIP and the Conservatives—And Populism and Euroscepticism. *Politics, 38*(3), 263–277.

Bergmann, E. (2018). *Conspiracy & Populism: The Politics of Misinformation.* Cham: Palgrave Macmillan.

Breeze, R. (2019). Positioning 'the People' and Its Enemies: Populism and Nationalism in AfD and UKIP. *Javnost—The Public, 26*(1), 89–104.

Cromby, J. (2019). The Myths of Brexit. *Journal for Applied Social Psychology, 29*, 56–66.

Ford, R., & Goodwin, M. (2014). Understanding UKIP: Identity, Social Change and the Left Behind. *The Political Quarterly, 85*(3), 277–284.

Reed, M. (2016). 'This Loopy Idea' an Analysis of UKIP's Social Media Discourse in Relation to Rurality and Climate Change. *Space and Polity, 20*(2), 226–241.

Rekawek, K. (2015). 'They Finished Second in 120 Seats:' UKIP and the Ongoing Revolt on the Right in the UK? *The Polish Quarterly of International Affairs, 24*(2), 163–178.

Taggart, P. (2017). Populism in Western Europe. In C. Rovira Kaltwasser, P. Taggart, P. Ochoa Espejo & P. Ostiguy (Eds.), *The Oxford Handbook of Populism* (pp. 248–263). Oxford: Oxford University Press.

Tournier-Sol, K. (2015). Reworking the Eurosceptic and Conservative Traditions into a Populist Narrative: UKIP's Winning Formula? *Journal of Common Market Studies, 53*(1), 140–156.

Tormey, S. (2020). Populism and the Pandemic: A Collaborative Report: United Kingdom. *POPULISMUS Interventions,* 7, 49–52.

CHAPTER 3

Spain: Is Ideology Back in Populist Discourse?

Jaume Magre, Lluís Medir, and Esther Pano

1 Introduction

Although in a representative and pluralistic democracy the task of the opposition is indispensable, so is the fact that the seriousness of the health situation in Spain has failed to impose the logic of consensus. Instead, what has prevailed is the logic of majority-opposition, which conservative parties have been able to take advantage of in a very effective way, especially VOX. The role of Unidas Podemos, the other great Spanish populist party, has been mediatised by its institutional position in the coalition Spanish government. Despite this different position, both have faced the COVID-19 pandemic leaving out populist argumentation and have, rather, enhanced the ideological content of their proposals. VOX has shown its radical-right-wing profile that, sometimes, they pretend to camouflage. And in the case of Unidas Podemos, they have been forced

J. Magre (✉) · E. Pano
Universitat de Barcelona and Fundació Carles Pi i Sunyer, Barcelona, Spain
e-mail: jmagre@ub.edu

L. Medir
Universitat de Barcelona, Barcelona, Spain

G. Bobba and N. Hubé (eds.), *Populism and the Politicization of the COVID-19 Crisis in Europe*,
https://doi.org/10.1007/978-3-030-66011-6_3

to emphasise their left-wing ideology to keep a profile of their own in the coalition government of which they are the minority partner.

The political construction of the discourse of both parties seems to be marked by the very evolution of the pandemic. Thus, we establish a chronology that begins with the break out of the health crisis and the approval of the state of constitutional alarm, followed by the strictest confinement period, and ending with the phase of de-scaling that has been described by the government with the concept of 'the new normality'.

2 Political Context

The year 2014 sees the emergence of the two main populist forces in Spain: Podemos and VOX. The appearance of both at the same time can be largely accounted for by the deep and prolonged economic crisis that had impacted on much of Spanish society and the realisation that the traditional mechanisms of political representation were incapable of channelling citizens' demands and indignation. This long economic crisis was particularly intense in the countries of southern Europe, and the way it was handled by certain political powers triggered shifts in attitudes away from the classic image of Spaniards' political culture, particularly due to a perceived lack of political efficacy or, to be more precise, political competence (Cordero and Montero 2015).

The two parties' brief electoral history runs from the 2014 European elections to the last time they competed: in the Spanish general elections of November 2019. A look at the timeline plotting the general elections they have taken part in shows them taking diverging paths. After initial electoral success, Podemos subsequently begins to show a marked downward trend: so much so that in less than five years it sees its electoral support fall by eight percentage points. It should not be forgotten that Podemos has for a long time been the institutional mouthpiece of the different social movements that arose in the early 2000s, and its gradual loss of electoral potential could be attributed to an inborn weakness (Torreblanca 2015; Galindo 2015). VOX, on the other hand, emerges when the most radical sector of the centre-right of the Partido Popular (People's Party, Spain's principal conservative party: PP) breaks away from this party. Its rise in the polls has been spectacular: going from a haul of 57,000 votes in 2015 to becoming the third political force in Spain four years later, with over three and a half million votes and 52 deputies in

Table 1 Main Spanish political parties (>5% in the last general election)

Political party	*November 2019 general election*		*2019 European election*	
	Vote shares (%)	*Seats*	*Vote shares (%)*	*Seats*
In power				
PSOE	27.7	120	32.8	20
UP	12.7	35	10.1	6
In opposition				
PP	20.6	88	20.1	12
VOX	14.9	52	6.2	3
C's	6.7	10	12.2	7

the Congreso de Diputados (Congress of Deputies, the Spanish Parliament). The same progression can be seen in the share of seats in the last four general elections. Podemos, in very few years, sees its parliamentary representation practically halved, while VOX goes from having no representatives in parliament to becoming the third political force in the chamber (Table 1).

Podemos's parliamentary results placed it in a weak negotiating position until the last elections, after which it made a deal with the winner, the Partido Socialista Obrero Español (Spanish Socialist Workers' Party: PSOE) and joined the government with a greater ministerial representation than its results warranted. Regarding Santiago Abascal's VOX party, it currently holds the key that lets the PP and Ciudadanos (Citizens: C's) govern in some autonomous communities, like Madrid and Andalusia, and in some municipalities. This gives an idea of its muscle in inter-party negotiations and power-sharing, but VOX's main victory lies in its ability to disrupt the political debate and force the PP into taking up more extreme ideological positions: something that this party would not have done without the parliamentary strength obtained by VOX in the last general elections.

The pandemic crisis coincides, moreover, with one of the most convulsive periods in recent years in politics and society, largely due to the judgement of the leaders of Catalonia's independence process, which has placed the focus of much of public debate on the territorial unity of the Spanish state. Additionally, to further complicate the situation, this debate has to be resolved in a context of political fragmentation in the party system that is much greater than normal in the Spanish electoral tradition. The result is easy to imagine: impossible coalitions and a centrifugal trend in the discourses of certain political parties.

3 COVID-19 Diffusion and Political Measures

Spain has suffered one of the worst COVID-19 outbreaks in the world. As the virus has continued to spread, Spain has become the country with the seventh highest number of both confirmed cases and of deaths. In June 2020 there were close to 300,000 cases, with 30,000 deaths (Fig. 1 and Table 2).

The Spanish public healthcare system has had to confront the crisis after a decade of austerity and low investment, which has placed health

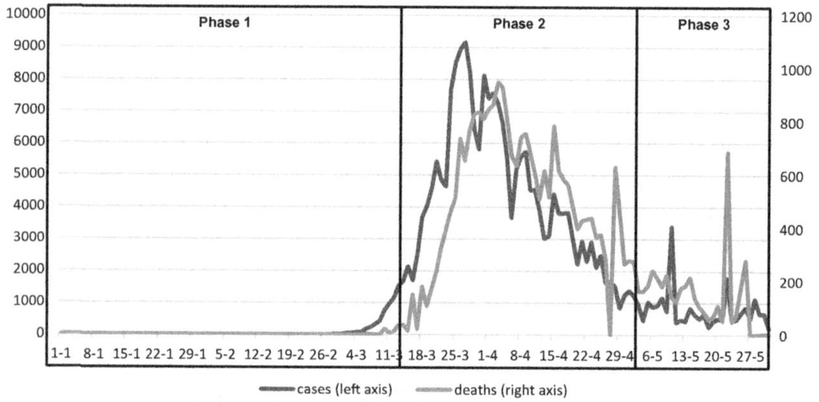

Fig. 1 Daily death toll and new cases in Spain (*Source* European Centre for Disease Prevention and Control. Phase 1: pre-COVID-19; Phase 2: spread and containment measures; Phase 3: contagion mitigation)

Table 2 COVID-19 pandemic in Spain

Cases	289,046
Total deaths	27,136
Total recovered	140,033
Cases per 1 M pop	6.182
Deaths per 1 M pop	580

Source www.worldometers.info/coronavirus/ (update 10/6/2020)

workers in a very precarious position. According to the European Commission report 'State of Health in the UE, 2019' (European Observatory on Health Systems and Policies 2019), Spain reduced its spending on health care by 5.3% between the 2008 crisis and 2015: almost 1% of its GDP. The number of hospital beds has fallen by a fifth since the start of the century: from 368 per 100,000 inhabitants in the year 2000 to 298 in 2015.

With the virus spreading rapidly, on 14 March 2020, the government declared a state of alarm pursuant to Article 116 of the Spanish constitution, and went on to extend it by two-week periods as many as six times. This state of alarm and the corresponding lockdown have been one of the longest and strictest of any European Union country. Perhaps for this reason, there has been some debate in Spain about restrictions on certain fundamental rights, mainly concerning the free movement of persons and business freedom.

In the midst of this political consternation, the principal measures taken by the government have focused on the labour market and social services, on the one hand, and on business incentives on the other. Regarding the first of these areas, apart from the suspension of evictions in the case of tenants who have lost their jobs due to COVID-19, the moratorium on mortgages, and the guaranteed supplies of electricity, gas and water during the crisis, the two most emblematic government measures have been the Temporary Lay-off Plans (ERTE) and the Minimum Living Income (IMV).

The ERTE is a mechanism that allows employment contracts to be suspended or working hours reduced temporarily, with the aim of avoiding redundancies during the health crisis and helping businesses, so that these can quickly resume their normal operations when the health situation allows. The Employment Ministry states that 3,386,785 workers were affected by an ERTE in Spain at the end of April 2020, which means a quarter of those signed up to the national insurance system. As for the IMV, this is a non-contributory Social Security benefit that guarantees a minimum income for those that would otherwise have none. It is defined as a subjective right of the citizenry: to be paid whenever the eligibility requirements are met, just like the right to a retirement pension or unemployment benefits. 255,000 citizens are expected to be eligible for the Minimum Living Income.

Despite all these measures, the OECD predicts that the Spanish economy will be the hardest–hit of all its members, with a contraction in GDP in 2020 of 14.4% and a 19.2% unemployment rate (OECD 2020). This bad economic forecast comes only a few years after the deep economic crisis of 2008 that plunged the country into a decade of austerity, unemployment and increased social inequality.

4 Populist Discourse at the Time of COVID-19

Just before the state of alarm was declared, Spanish politics was going through a period of high political tension, marked by constant partisan conflict. The COVID-19 pandemic has only served to exacerbate this confrontation. Spanish citizens are aware of this and over 80% of them describe the situation as inflamed, according to data from the 'Barometer' of the Centre for Sociological Research (CIS), and a quarter regard Santiago Abascal and his VOX party as the main sources of this tension. Their reactions are similar when assessing the role of the opposition during the response to the pandemic: only 10% of the total population of Spain approve of the stance taken up by VOX and its main leader Santiago Abascal during the months of lockdown.

The latter's opposition, according to experts in political communication, is unequalled in its intensity and use of disinformation techniques to discredit the Spanish government and certain political organisations. In fact, this is not the first time VOX has been accused of disinformation. The European Commission's security commissioner, Julian King, named VOX on 14 June 2019 as an example of disinformation and rumour-peddling on social media.

VOX's permanent confrontation with the executive seems to come from a wish to take on the role of 'national opposition' and monopolise protests against the government. In this, it is favoured by the current political climate, as the party system has been in a state of upheaval for some time. C's is swerving towards the political centre and exploring a possible deal with the executive, while the PP is manoeuvring to prevent its criticism of President Sánchez from eroding its image as a 'party of state'.[1] VOX, therefore, has considerable room for manoeuvre towards achieving its wish, fighting for the ideological monopoly of the Spanish right and making the PP change political course. In the end, what is in dispute is the post-pandemic narrative and, here, VOX has shown itself

[1] Casals, X., VOX i la Covid-19. *El Periódico*, 10/5/2020.

to be more than capable of setting the public agenda and the terms of debate. The unexpected result of this new position is that the intensity, harshness and disproportionality of its criticism of the government give it almost the appearance of an anti-establishment party.

The new institutional role of Unidas Podemos (United We Can: UP)—a member of the governing coalition with the PSOE since the general elections of November 2019—implies a need for solidarity between the members of the executive and, therefore, its public profile has been much lower during the pandemic, which reached Spain within only three months of their taking office. Whatever the case, the fact that four ministries controlled by the PSOE (Health, Interior, Defence and Transport) were placed in charge of managing the health crisis has pushed UP into the background, so it has tried to regain the political limelight through two different strategies: firstly by presenting itself before the public as being in charge of the so-called social shield (the set of social measures to protect the most vulnerable groups against COVID) and, secondly, by taking public responsibility for rebutting the arguments of the nativist radical right. In other words, it could be said that the populist characteristics of UP are slowly fading away and it is taking on board the principles of a traditional party of the European left. This would explain the obsession with avoiding at all costs the solutions adopted in the 2008 economic crisis, which led to greater inequality, a huge growth in unemployment and widespread poverty across the population (Montero's Twitter account 17/4/2020; Montero's Twitter account 1/5/2020; Iglesias's Twitter account 27/3/2020).

To sum up, here we have two very different strategies for making political use of the COVID-19 pandemic. In the case of VOX, the strategic burden of defending the nation has made it a practically anti-establishment party. On the other hand, UP is conditioned by its institutional role as part of the governing coalition, which has probably lent weight to its identity as a party of the left to the detriment of its populist tendencies.

The question now is how these populist organisations have adapted their discourse during the pandemic. As far as VOX is concerned, although it maintains the main arguments of nativist populism that characterise it, what the COVID-19 pandemic has brought to light is this organisation's radical-right positions. That is to say, while the common thread running through the pronouncements of its main leaders continues to be the idea of rescuing the nation from those who are perverting and damaging it—currently the government and the 'Chavist communists' of UP—it is also true that populist rhetoric does not appear directly in VOX's discourse: it could have adopted an anti-science discourse or held up the health workers and the security forces as an example to shame the political elites who left them to their fate, but it has not done so. VOX is more interested in disrupting the party system and appearing as the true national defender of the people against the government. Accordingly, it has berated the executive, accusing it of using the pandemic, now that Spaniards' guard is down, as an excuse to impose a totalitarian regime through a state of emergency disguised as a (less drastic) state of alarm (Abascal's Twitter account, 19/5/2020; Olona's Twitter account, 11/3/2020). As evidence of this, it points to what it sees as a disproportionate restriction of fundamental rights: mainly personal freedom of movement, business freedom and freedom of worship or assembly, using words like 'totalitarian government', 'dictatorship', 'genocide' and 'communism', and clamouring for 'liberty' and an end to the lockdown. And it goes even further. According to VOX, the government's actions have amounted to an attack on the right to life, since euthanasia, which is illegal in Spain, has been practised with extreme ferocity on elderly persons in care homes. VOX has gone on to bring criminal proceedings (a *querella*) against the executive before the Supreme Court, for crimes of serious imprudence resulting in death (Monasterio's Twitter account 18/5/2020).

The remainder of VOX's discourse consists of nativist nationalism. National and cultural identity as an element of resistance to national, foreign and supra-national elites (De Cleen 2017) appears in most of the speeches made by the organisation's leaders in parliament and in public. It should come as no surprise, therefore, that its Secretary General for Organisation, Ortega Smith, has referred to '*Spanish antibodies*' as a way to combat '*those damned Chinese viruses*'. VOX's striking nationalism has remained intact throughout the pandemic.

In fact, the hard-hitting spread of the pandemic through Spain has allowed it to double down on its claims about global insecurity, borders, immigration, economic protectionism, national unity and centralised decision-making, providing a justification for its highly publicised ideological principles (Fernández 2020).

The situation of UP is different. Although the path taken by this political organisation leads to its consolidation as a left-wing party, this does not mean to say that it has completely abandoned the populist ideas that marked its origins. Ultimately, the two souls that have been present in the party since its foundation continue to exist and compete. This would explain why, at the height of the pandemic, it has endorsed the campaigns against the monarchy and former king Juan Carlos I and against the Deep State.

5 The Politicization of COVID-19 Issue by Populists

This section traces the development of the populist discourse in Spain, highlighting the process by which VOX and Podemos construct their position on management of the pandemic. The process begins with the exploding health crisis and the ensuing declaration of a state of alarm under the Constitution, continues with the period of strict lockdown and ends with the de-escalation phase and what the government terms the 'new normality'.

The first phase of politicization lasted from the healthcare disaster in early March to the declaration of a state of alarm under the Constitution in mid-March. VOX and Podemos view the problem through their own lenses.

Although VOX clashes with the government from the very start of the pandemic, it is visibly disconcerted by the seriousness of the health situation, along with the rest of the Spanish political class. The institutional policy it adopts in those early days is nothing like the one it will pursue later: it does not oppose the government's state of alarm declaration on 14 March and even votes in favour of its first extension on 28 March. From then on, however, it votes against all subsequent extensions of the state of alarm, radically opposing the strict stay-at-home lockdown that is initially enforced in Spain.

At this early stage, VOX's approach is to send out messages of support for health workers and security forces, mixed in with patriotic slogans. VOX's messages stray very little from the official discourse at the time: transmitting bewilderment, fear, a sense of unreality and of being in the midst of events of great significance, and, at the same time calling for unity, responsibility and teamwork and praising the health workers (Fernández 2020). The line VOX takes is to unreservedly support the police and the health workers, trying to insert patriotic slogans into its messages of encouragement, while at the same time resorting to the classic resources of populism, appealing to an intact, all-powerful people. '*[...]*

the determination of the Spanish people to continue advancing is our best asset. The people have always stepped up in the end when the institutions have failed' (Abascal's Twitter account, 14/3/2020).

Meanwhile, Podemos, as a minority member of the first coalition government in Spain's recent democratic history, finds itself in an ambivalent position at that early stage: without denying the seriousness of the health situation and the need to take urgent, drastic measures, it seems to (mildly) disapprove of a constitutional state of alarm that excessively curtails fundamental rights and even involves the military to a high degree.

This leads to friction between PSOE ministers and Podemos government members. The disagreement is basically about the financial impact of the lockdown on workers and means that a meeting over seven hours long was needed for the government to pass the state of alarm.[2] In that phase, Podemos begins to define the health crisis also in terms of social protection for the worst-hit citizens.

During the second phase, the management of the pandemic grows stricter and restrictions on fundamental rights and the economic deterioration increase. It is in this second phase that VOX culminates the switch to a strategy of hounding the government and the centralised medical command to destruction. It starts taking a more critical stance, focusing on the government's lack of foresight, the shortages of medical supplies, the thronged feminist demonstrations held on 8 March, and the high numbers of infections and deaths. This means abandoning all traces of the minimal institutional loyalty shown up to that point and ruthlessly switching to ferocious attacks on the coalition government's performance.

The result of this is that during most of the lockdown it is VOX that acts as the real opposition to the government. VOX's policy of all-out criticism of the government's handling of the crisis is clearly aimed at wearing down the PP, the dominant centre-right party in the chamber, taking advantage of the latter's role as a 'party of state' that votes on three consecutive occasions to extend the state of alarm and abstains in the fourth vote, despite having kept up a consistently critical stance. Subsequently, the PP joins VOX in voting against extending the state of alarm on three further occasions.

[2] Las divergencias entre el PSOE y UP sobre el plan de choque económico alargan el Consejo de ministros. *El Pais*, 14/3/2020.

The rationale behind VOX's policy of criticising the handling of the crisis is basically this: the exceptionally bad handling of the crisis in Spain deserves exceptionally harsh criticism (Fernández 2020). In its discourse, VOX claims that responsibility for the pandemic and the chaotic health-care situation lies with the government's decision-making. The words that stand out the most in its discourse in this period are irresponsibility, ideology, improvisation, incompetence and bad management: '… *we see a government that is unprepared to cope with the challenges to health and the economy posed by a pandemic*', '*recklessly putting health workers in danger*', '*conducting too few tests*', '*allowing an alarming shortage of masks*'.

VOX's metamorphosis with regard to the other radical-right parties in Europe begins in the last week of March, when, after criticising the executive's handling of the crisis, it demands the government's resignation. This initiates an escalation that leads Santiago Abascal's party to call for *caceroladas* (pot-banging protests) in the name of freedom and to fight on several fronts to bring down the coalition government. In this phase, it goes back to its roots as a political and civil spearhead against the 'social-communist government'.

At the same time, Podemos completely abandons any hint of criticism of the government's performance to concentrate on a discourse of protection for the most underprivileged sectors of society. While the actual handling of the health crisis remains in the hands of PSOE ministers, Podemos ministers get on with building the 'social shield' narrative. Podemos's public discourse hinges on two fundamental components: social protection, on the one hand, and attacking the opposition from VOX and the PP, to a lesser extent.

As for the first of these, Podemos takes on the job of designing and defending a socially just way out of the crisis, focusing on the reconstruction of the welfare state, fair taxation and the recovery of the public sector as the basis for economic and social recovery. In this phase, it lays particular emphasis on the idea that the weight of the economic crisis should not be borne by the disadvantaged and the working class, as was the case in the 2008 financial crisis (Iglesias's Twitter account, 14/5/2020; 17/5/2020; 12/5/2020).

At the same time, it seems to specialise in knife-wielding for the government, mainly against the attacks coming from VOX. 'The extreme right is irritated by democracy and social justice' (Montero's Twitter account, 18/6/2020), 'VOX would like to stage a coup d'état, but they don't dare to'.[3] The PP is moving further and further away from Spain and from being a useful opposition' (Iglesias's Twitter account, 10/6/2020). However, in accusing the opposition of lack of cooperation and disloyalty, its rhetoric is not particularly populist in nature.

Having controlled the first wave of the health crisis, Spain finally entered in the third phase when the government ends the state of alarm and places the management of the post-pandemic situation back in the hands of the Autonomous Communities.

In this scenario, VOX fades into the background as the opposition to the government, since the PP sticks to its policy of repeatedly disputing the government's management of health care. This means that VOX will now turn all its attention from health care to the parliamentary electoral campaigns in the Basque Country and Galicia, taking aim at the Basque Nationalist Party—one of the government's main parliamentary supporters—at Podemos (Abascal's Twitter account, 28/6/2020), and at the Galician PP. In other words, it goes back to its classic strategy of confronting peripheral nationalisms in Spain, apparently assuming it has capitalised fully on its healthcare stance.

Podemos, meanwhile, continues to showcase its social approach to managing the crisis and the solidity of the coalition government, and forcefully renews its criticisms of the performance of conservative parties wherever these have been in power: 'It's indecent that, when the main lesson to be drawn from the pandemic is the need to take better care of public health services and their workers, wherever the PP is in charge it continues to privatise hospital services, as they're doing in Madrid. They have learned nothing' (Iglesias's Twitter account, 24/6/2020).

6 Conclusion

The results of the survey Public Opinion in Times of COVID-19, commissioned by the European Parliament, reveal Spaniards to be the European citizens who are the most critical of their government's handling of the COVID-19 health crisis. Aside from the government's performance in this regard, the fact that it is the worst rated also reflects the political tension that has filled Spain during the months of lockdown:

[3] Iglesias admite su salida de tono en la Comisión de reconstrucción pero subraya que dijo la verdad. *Diario ABC*, 29/5/2020.

a tension that in recent years has led to changes of government following major political, social and economic crises.

Events like the public opposition to the Iraq war in 2002, the 11 M terrorist attacks in 2004, the economic crisis in 2008 and the motion of censure against President Rajoy in 2018 were largely responsible for ousting the party in government. VOX has sensed this opportunity and has decided to use the pandemic to direct fierce criticism at the Spanish government, to the point of becoming practically an anti-establishment party. Podemos's role is obviously conditioned by its institutional position as part of the Spanish government. This would explain why, at one point, the Secretary for Organisation of UP declared that 'after almost a hundred days of the state of alarm, we can look around at the international scene and conclude that the coalition government has done the right thing' (Echenique's Twitter account, 21/6/2020).

While the two parties have adopted differing strategies towards the government's performance, there are similarities between them, however, regarding the populist component in their messaging. In response to the COVID-19 pandemic, both have discarded their populist standpoints to a great extent and, instead, highlighted the ideological content of their proposals. Not once have they resorted to the anti-science and anti-expert discourse that is so typical of these types of organisations, nor have they used the health workers as a judgemental people-versus-political-class symbol. VOX, to the contrary, has adopted the role of 'national opposition' to the government of Spain and has exhibited the radical-right profile that it had previously kept hidden. The intention is to capitalise on the pandemic to disrupt the party system and emerge as the representative of a certain Spanish right. As for UP, it has had to accentuate its left-wing component to maintain a distinct profile as a minority member of the coalition government. This is the main reason why it has claimed to be the force behind the so-called social shield and its greatest defender.

Ultimately, it is not easy to gauge how much both parties' strategies will affect voting in the general elections. In fact, the first round has already taken place, in July 2020, a month after the lockdown: two of the historical Autonomous Communities—Galicia and the Basque Country—held elections to their own parliaments. The results reveal that the fall in electoral support that Podemos has been suffering since 2015 still continues: never has it had so much power and so few votes. VOX, on the other hand, has held steady in elections that were never likely to give it a boost. There is no causal link of any kind between the position it held during the pandemic and the results obtained in Autonomous-Community elections, but these results do hint at how it will approach the elections to the Spanish Parliament.

References

Cordero, G., & Montero, J. R. (2015). Against Bipartyism, Towards Dealignment? The 2014 European Election in Spain. *South European Society and Politics*, *20*(3), 357–379.

De Cleen, B. (2017). Populism and Nationalism. In C. Rovira, P. Taggart, P. Ochoa, & P. Osiguy (Eds.), *The Oxford Handbook of Populism*. Oxford: Oxford University Press.

European Observatory on Health Systems and Policies. (2019). State of Health in the UE.

Fernández, G. (2020, May 28). La venezuelización de VOX durante la pandemia. *La U. Revista de cultura y pensamiento*.

Galindo, J. (2015). Movilización social y representación política en España: de los indignados a Podemos. In A. Minnaert & E. Gustavo (Eds.), *Democracia participativa e izquierda. Logros, contradicciones y desafíos*. Fundación Friedrich Ebert.

OECD. (2020). OECD Economic Outlook.

Torreblanca, I. (2015). *Asaltar los cielos. Podemos o la política después de la crisis*. Barcelona: Debate.

CHAPTER 4

Italy: Populist in the Mirror, (De)Politicizing the COVID-19 from Government and Opposition

Arturo Bertero and Antonella Seddone

1 Introduction

The identification of a pandemic outbreak in Italy at the end of February 2020 was unanticipated. Despite the concern for what was happening in the Hubei province, coronavirus disease 2019 (COVID-19) was considered specifically a 'Chinese problem'. This was an incorrect assumption. Even when the first Italian cases were diagnosed, there was still no awareness of the seriousness of the upcoming emergency. Italian politics was unprepared for this shock and consequently had to redefine its strategies. In this respect, being in opposition or in government determined different opportunities and challenges. This chapter investigated the diverse role played by the two most prominent Italian populist parties in the first four months of the emergency: the League (Lega) and the Five

A. Bertero (✉) · A. Seddone
Department of Cultures, Politics and Society, University of Turin, Turin, Italy
e-mail: arturo.bertero@edu.unito.it

G. Bobba and N. Hubé (eds.), *Populism and the Politicization of the COVID-19 Crisis in Europe*,
https://doi.org/10.1007/978-3-030-66011-6_4

Star Movement (M5S, Movimento 5 Stelle). The League attempted to adapt to the emergency to its usual populist strongholds. Conversely, the M5S, as a government party, emphasised its responsiveness by appealing for national unity and claiming the ownership for those governmental action providing direct support to citizens.

2 Political Context

Italy has been described as the 'promised land' of populism (Tarchi 2015) or as its 'breeding ground' (Bobba and Legnante 2016) because of the durable success of its populist parties. The emergence of the Northern League (LN, Lega Nord) in the late 1980s and the unexpected performance of Berlusconi at the head of Go Italy (FI, Forza Italia) in the early 1990s represented the first steps of populism's recent history in Italy. The success of the M5S since 2013 has expanded the variety of populism, including parties not belonging to the right. Although in the past, Berlusconi has been described as the champion of the Italian 'neoliberal populism' (Mudde and Rovira Kaltvasser 2017), in the last few years, he adopted less populist positions (Mazzoleni and Bracciale 2018; see also 2019 Chapel Hill expert survey) to the extent of describing himself as the only opponent of the populist threat during the 2018 general elections (Roncarolo and Cremonesi 2019).[1] Currently, the M5S and the League are indisputably not only the two most important populist parties but also amongst the main key players in Italian politics. Although in 2018 they supported a coalition government together, they are profoundly different in terms of political histories, political programmes and belongingness in varieties of populism.

The M5S was formally founded in 2009 by Beppe Grillo, an Italian comedian, and the late web entrepreneur Gianroberto Casaleggio. The 2013 Italian general election was a turning point for the party. In its first national electoral campaign, it had striking success: Grillo's anti-political style resonated well with Italians' deep distrust for the political class. A quarter of Italian voters (25.56%) cast their ballot for the M5S that entered the Italian Parliament as an opposition party. The transformation of Grillo's movement into a proper institutional political actor

[1] Notably, a new right-wing party, Fratelli d'Italia (FDI, Brothers of Italy), is probably qualified to be called a populist. However, considering the lesser relevance than of the M5S and the League, it was not included in this chapter because of space constraints.

was completed during the 2013–2018 legislature. In 2018, the M5S approached the Italian elections as an experienced political party ready to take up posts in government. After the step back of its founder, the M5S party membership formally appointed Luigi Di Maio as the new leader of the movement with full responsibility for leading the party through the 2018 election campaign.[2] The result was gratifying: the party was confirmed as Italy's most popular with 32.7% of the vote. During this period, the M5S has combined its clear anti-establishment rhetoric with a blurry ideological positioning. Although initially the movement espoused a vaguely leftist ideology (D'Alimonte 2019: 120), after its success in the 2013 general election (see Tronconi 2015), the party started to shift its positioning on the political spectrum. The blurring of its left–right positioning has caused several political scholars to describe the party as having a post-ideological profile that is 'beyond left and right classification' (Tarchi 2015).

The League is the heir of the Northern League, an ethno-regionalist party founded by the charismatic figure of Umberto Bossi who promoted secessionist or federalist policies to favour Northern regions (Albertazzi and McDonnell 2010). In 2013, major changes in the party organisation led to the appointment of a new leader, Matteo Salvini. This shift at the head of the party entailed an ideological redefinition. Whilst Bossi's LN was right-leaning and regionally based, Salvini's League is a staunchly far-right populist party. As the party moved onto the national level, patriotism replaced regionalism, and the European Union (EU) and immigrants replaced Rome and Southern Italians as the people's enemy (D'Alimonte 2019: 122). The party has increasingly focused on immigration, national identity and law and order issues (Albertazzi et al. 2018; Bobba 2019). This new ideological stance and Salvini's enthusiastic leadership have been highly rewarded by voters making the League the first party in the centre-right field.

After a brief interlude where together the M5S and the League supported the first Conte government, in August 2019, Salvini withdrew his support while the M5S decided to back a second Conte government

[2] It is necessary to mention that on January 22, 2020, following the resignation of Luigi Di Maio as political head of the M5S, Vito Crimi takes over the leadership of the party on an interim basis. Luigi di Maio remains in any case the most prominent and relevant representative of the M5S due to his government role as Minister of Foreign Affairs.

Table 1 Main Italian political parties (>5% in the last General election)

Political party	*General election 2018*		*European Election 2019*	
	Vote shares	*Seats*	*Vote shares*	*Seats*
In power				
Five Star Movement	32.7	133	17.1	14
Democratic Party	18.8	86	22.7	19
In opposition				
The League	17.4	73	34.3	29
Go Italy	14.0	59	8.8	7

with the left-wing Partito Democratico (Democratic Party). The COVID-19 crisis finds the two parties in a mirror situation: the M5S is in power but with a low approval rate; the League is instead in opposition but with a growing number of voters (Table 1).

3 COVID-19 Diffusion and Political Measures

In Italy, there was no clue regarding the risk of an actual outbreak of the pandemic, during the *first phase*. The first measures taken by the Italian national government in the prevention of a possible spread of the COVID-19 within the country were issued in January. After the notice regarding a pandemic hitting the Hubei province, the World Health Organization as well as the European Centre for Disease Prevention and Control put out a warning but still indicating a moderate risk of actual contagion across the European countries. The Italian government reacted through the establishment of a dedicated task force dealing with a possible health emergency.[3] In the absence of full-blown cases, the government's actions focused mainly on monitoring the transport of passengers and goods between Italy and China. At the end of January, after two Chinese tourists in Rome were diagnosed positive to the infection, the Minister of Health disposed the block of all flights from China. Furthermore, since all the (few) diagnosed cases had a strong and direct connection with China, the national government limited the use of diagnostic swabs only to patients who had contact with the Chinese outbreak. Basically, during

[3] All the measures taken by the Italian government are available here: http://www.governo.it/it/coronavirus (last accessed: June 2020).

this pre-COVID-19 phase, the risk of an actual outbreak in Italy was perceived as remote, simply requiring prevention and monitoring.

However, very suddenly, Italy entered a *second phase*, when the presence of the virus was overt and the increasing contagion rates, as well as the pressure on the health system, revealed the very nature of the pandemic emergency. It was precisely the absence of recent contact with China that triggered the alarm, when on 21 February, a young patient was diagnosed positive for COVID-19 in a small village, just outside Milan. A few days later, other patients were hospitalised in the nearby area with symptoms consistent with COVID-19; the same happened in a small centre in the Veneto region. COVID-19 was no more only a Chinese problem. Because of the identification of two different outbreaks in Northern Italy, the government issued the first of an incremental set of measures aimed to contain the contagion. On 24 February, two red zones limited to the municipalities involved in the infection were identified, and the limitation of movement and the closure of non-essential services were lifted.[4] In about a week, the daily number of infected individuals doubled, and the pressure on hospitals and intensive care units increased leading the government to issue a second set of measures. On 1 March, the red zone was extended including most of the provinces of Northern Italy.[5] Considering the increasing pressure over the hospitals and intensive care units, as well as the scarcity of diagnostic swabs and the limited supply of individual protection devices to health workers, the national government on 11 March 2020, decided to tighten the lockdown measures extending them to all the Italian territory.[6] Particularly, the virus was hitting Northern Italy, but contagion cases were determined all over the country. A nationwide closure was specifically decided to prevent Southern regions—with structural deficits in health facilities—from rising contagion rates. All teaching activities in schools and universities were suspended, and bars, restaurants and shops except for those providing essential services (like food stores and pharmacies) were closed. Ten days later, due to the increasing contagion rate and the response to pressure

[4] Decree *Dpcm 23 febbraio 2020*.

[5] Decree *Dpcm 1 marzo 2020*.

[6] Decree *Dpcm 11 marzo 2020*.

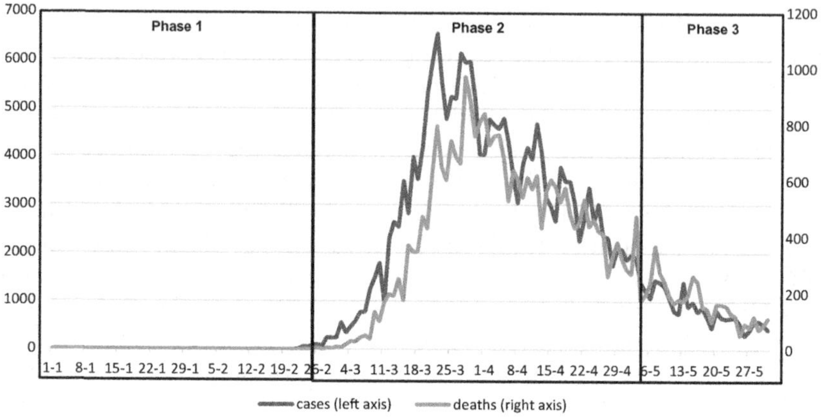

Fig. 1 Daily death toll and new cases in Italy (*Source* European Centre for Disease Prevention and Control. Phase 1: pre-COVID-19; Phase 2: spread and containment measures; Phase 3: contagion mitigation)

from unions concerned about the safety of workers, the national government decided to further intensify the lockdown by shutting down all non-necessary businesses and industries.

The *third phase* coincides with the mitigation of contagion, ensuing the lockdown end and the gradual reopening of the economic and production activities within the country. Formally, the closure was expected to end on 13 April, but it eventually came about ending on 4 May. Whilst the movement across regions was still forbidden, citizens were allowed to leave their homes to their visit relatives. Industrial plants, shops, bars and restaurants were allowed to open. Since 3 June, movement across regions was able to return to a semi-normal situation. Whilst schools and universities were still closed, the other activities gradually returned to normal, although limitations concerning social distancing remained (Fig. 1 and Table 2).

4 Populist Discourse at the Time of COVID-19

The M5S and the League faced the period of the COVID-19 pandemic from opposite institutional positions with different constraints and opportunities. As a major government party, the Movement was called to take prompt decisions to respond to the crisis; in opposition, the League

Table 2 COVID-19 pandemic in Italy

Cases	235,561
Total death	34,043
Total recovered	168,646
Cases for 1 M pop	3896
Deaths for 1M pop	563

Source https://www.worldometers.info/coronavirus/ (update 10/6/2020)

continued to criticise the government, although its flagship proposals appeared undermined in a political field entirely absorbed by the health crisis. These two general patterns differently impacted on their populist discourse and on the variation of the key elements within it.

The M5S usually adopts a Manichean vision of society and refers to 'the people' as the honest citizens who are committed to fighting the corrupt system. During the pandemic, this view slightly changed becoming more inclusive and less based on divisive issues: all the Italians have to be protected and saved, and politics should be united as well for facing such a situation. This attitude was evident in several Di Maio's statements highly sympathetic with the Italians: '*I read you and understand all your difficulties. This damned virus has upset our days, our lives, but we are reacting and this is important. [...] Let's prove we are a great people*' (Di Maio's Facebook page, 29/03/20). The crisis also allows the Movement to reiterate the relevance of citizenship income by stating that '*politics must support its people, starting with the weakest, those who have lost their smiles and suffer for no faults of their own*' (Di Maio's interview, Guerra e Pace, 17/04/20, *TV2000*). Likewise, the League shown an inclusive view of the people. Indeed, Salvini empathized with the Italians fuelling their pride. However, 'the people' is always defined in contrast with the elites or the outgroups. In these respects, the pandemic crisis did not change much the way the League exalted the sovereignty of the Italian State or his leader claimed to represent and defend the Italian people.

Certainly, the arguments used by the League for blaming 'the elites' have changed. Although the targeted elites are still the same—the Italian ruling class and the EU—the list of charges has been updated. The uncertain situation offered an opportunity to blame the government for whatever. Particularly, it was accused of endangering the Italian people by being incompetent in the management of the health emergency: in January, the League protested that Italy had not closed its borders before the outbreak of the pandemic, whilst in Easter (6 April) the stated measures had to be relaxed to allow, for example, people to go to church.[7] Similarly, all the government efforts made for responding to the economic crisis were considered systematically insufficient. In this respect, Salvini often report individual stories of people in need (i.e. '*I have the mailbox, Messenger, WhatsApp and mobile phone full of messages from Italians—merchants, entrepreneurs, self-employed, freelancers, families and workers in general—who despite government decrees and promises have not yet received a euro refund*', Salvini's Facebook page, 08/04/20). The second favourite target of the League, the EU institutions, is usually accused of being inadequate and serving the interests of other countries. In the light of the COVID-19 crisis, these accusations are specified in the delay of the EU reaction to the pandemic and then shifted especially on the European Stability Mechanism (ESM), claimed as conceived at the detriment of the Italian people ('*ESM approved: outside the law, dictature in the name of the virus [...] Since 1989 Italy has paid 140 billion to Europe, now to borrow 35 billion we have to accept a system of a legalized loan sharking system*'[8]). Although anti-elitism is a central feature of the M5S discourse, the targeted elites changed during the crisis. The issue of corruption and the wasting of public funds are temporarily set aside. In the initial phase of the pandemic, Di Maio blamed the international media—one of the traditional targets of the Movement—for creating a climate of fear and hatred towards Italy. Moreover, some critics were moved towards the EU. Unlike what Salvini did (and the Movement too in the past), these were not attacks but rather firm stances on the need for economic and financial aid to resolve the crisis ('*We are a people who have always given to the European Union, now is the time to receive. As Italy today we are fighting a war against an invisible enemy and Europe must help us*' Di Maio's interview, TG1, 26/03/20). Notably, this attempt at dialogue with an archetypal elite such as the EU is probably strategic, mainly due to the M5S's position in power and Di Maio's role as foreign minister. The need to offer a responsive and effective image determined also the reframe of the M5S's indulgence with anti-science claims.

[7] M. Cremonesi, Riaprire le chiese a Pasqua? Tutti contro Salvini (cattolici compresi). *Corriere della Sera*, 05/04/20.

[8] Eurogruppo, Salvini: 'C'è il Mes, così è ipoteca sul futuro'. Meloni: 'Vincono Germania e Olanda'. *Il Messaggero*, 09/04/20.

Lining up with the government coalition's partner, indeed, the Movement is now committed and supportive of science. Consequently, those formerly labelled as elites—such as experts, pharmaceutical industries and mainstream scientists generally—became swiftly the only trustworthy referents leading the government actions against the virus (i.e. '*There is a scientific committee that will tell the government when we can return to normality*'[9]). This is particularly relevant because, on the other side, Salvini has exploited this populist argument by winking more than once to conspiracy theories about the origin of the virus and effective treatment methods against COVID-19 kept hidden by pharmaceutical companies (Salvini's Twitter account, 05/05/20).

The third element of populism—'the outgroups'—only applies to the League. The M5S, even when in government with the League, never really developed anti-migrant or discriminatory positions towards ethnic-religious minorities or the LGBT community. By contrast, as containment measures became more severe, Salvini insisted on the frame of the 'uncontrolled immigration'. He counterposed the honest and law-abiding Italian people to irregular migrants and foreign drug dealers, committing crimes or landing without any health control ('*The government deploys Army and Police to control and fine Italians, but illegal immigrants continue to land...*'. Salvini's Twitter account, 27/03/20). This element, particularly in its 'law and order' variant, was weakened in the lockdown phase when the entire population was asked to stay at home and, consequently, the volume of common crimes (such as theft, robbery and drug dealing) decreased by 64%.[10]

5 The Politicization of COVID-19 Issue by Populists

The differences in how the two populist parties 'name, blame and claim' (Felstiner et al. 1980) of the health crisis relate mainly to the different roles played within the political landscape.

In the *emergence phase*, precisely when the COVID-19 pandemic appeared just as a Chinese problem, the League immediately recognised

[9] Di Maio, riaprire? Ce lo diranno esperti. *ANSA*, 01/04/20.

[10] Grignetti, F. Tutti a casa per il coronavirus, crollano i reati del 64%. *La Stampa*, 20/03/20.

the issue as a ground for applying its usual populist rhetoric. The *naming* of the virus points at the risk of contagion and the safeguard of Italian people. However, the League entered the issue in the political debate as one of the political arms to accuse the government. In this regard, it was used to revolve around the immigration problem, emphasising the need to close the border to foreign arrivals (i.e. '*Given that the Coronavirus emergency unfortunately is still high and concerning, a serious government should INTENSIFY controls on those arriving in Italy rather than proposing a policy for opening seaports*' Salvini's Facebook page, 21/02/20).

The M5S, given its role in government, coped with the pandemic emergency differently. The M5S and the government as a whole adopted the strategy of delaying the politicization of the issue by resorting to technical and scientific knowledge. The issue is thus addressed in terms of responsive actions for protecting Italian people from the COVID-19 contagion. The M5S named the COVID-19 issue as political only when the Italians outbreak was identified and the contagion rate certified the seriousness of the epidemic. Confronted with the growing pressure over the health system, the Movement changed its approach by asking other political parties for national unity and justifying the need for severe containment measures adopted as the only possible solution (i.e. *the state in all its parts is working hard to cope with the Coronavirus epidemic. And I believe that in these moments it is necessary to show unity and compactness [...] a politics with sense of responsibility is needed, which must look each other in the eye and think first of all about the interest of the citizens*).[11]

Lockdown measures resulted in a decreased pressure on intensive care units and concerns about the endurance of the health system. It is precisely at this moment that the League shifted into the *confrontation phase*, blaming the EU and national government for the management of the emergency. As the contagions grew, the short- and long-term consequences of the crisis became increasingly evident both in social and economic respects. The EU is accused of being silent or making vague promises whilst '*a lot of money is needed, immediately*' (Salvini's Facebook page 10/03/20). Regarding the national government, the nature of the League criticism is less definite. The seriousness of the pandemic impeded an open criticism over the lockdown measures. Therefore, the field of

[11] Coronavirus, Di Maio: 'Bisogna mostrare unità e compattezza'. *Adnkronos*, 21/02/20.

battle was organised around the economic consequences of the emergency and the lack of adequate economic support for citizens. However, identifying a specific issue on which the League had proved the ownership is difficult. Rather, the party focused its attention on a wide list of claims (and grievances), ranging from the incapability of the national government to provide adequate support for regional health systems to the bureaucratic constraints set by the government measures in support of citizens facing economic difficulties due to the lockdown. Similarly, the government was blamed for its leniency (and alleged interest) towards the ESM, perceived as an attempt from the EU institutions to force Italy to austerity policies and reforms (*'If they can find 15 billion for Africa and to Italy they can only say 'Either you get the ESM, putting yourself in a cage, or there is nothing for you'. If so, I understand those mayors who lowered the flag of Europe, of an institution that is proving to be aloof. This is not the European Union, it's the German Union'*. Salvini's Facebook page, 08/04/20).

The *confrontation phase* was instead addressed through a passive strategy by the M5S, having little chance of blaming anyone. The political scope of the measures implemented by the government was weakened and immediately justified by the technical–scientific committee of the Civil Protection Department. However, after the European Central Bank refused to issue extraordinary measures in support of countries suffering from financial speculation due to the pandemic, the M5S—along with other government parties—engaged in a heated debate with the EU institutions that marked the culmination of this phase. Controversies were healed only after the official commitment of the Head of the EU Commission to provide financial assistance to countries, easing the EU financial requirements and launching a series of funding schemes for economic recovery. The opening of the EU on this field, particularly regarding flexibility over the domestic budget, was claimed to be a success for the government and again the M5S has softened its traditional diffidence over the EU.[12]

As pertains to the *managing phase* of the COVID-19 issue, we could identify two different levels of policy interventions. The first one relates to the measures aimed to contain the contagion spread. The second one

[12] D'Argenio, A., Coronavirus, Von der Leyen: 'La Ue deve scusarsi con l'Italia'. *la Repubblica*, 16/04/20.

focuses on the consequences at the economic level. Indeed, the lockdown measures implied a stop to industrial production along with a dramatic fall in consumers spending, determining a negative outlook for the Italian economy with an expected collapse of the Italian GDP for 2020. Gradually, as the contagion rate started to decrease, particularly in Southern regions, the concerns for the health risk shifted on the economic dimension, putting the latter at the core of the political agenda. Besides the support for companies and enterprises, further measures were delivered. Since the beginning of the emergency, the government suspended all ongoing layoff procedures, introducing a mechanism of redundancy funds paid directly with public money. These measures were integrated with actions in support of freelancers and those categories of workers lacking social and economic protection. Incidentally, these measures were in line with the cornerstone of the original M5S's policy platform—the basic income. Easily, the party was able to claim ownership. Regarding the League, triggering the politicization of the COVID-19 emergency becomes quite arduous, and the party failed in getting the ownership of a recognisable topic. Relying on the usual populist claims—blaming migrants and the EU elites—was not sufficient to set the agenda during the health crisis, even less during the *managing phase* when policy proposals were under discussion. Lacking a recognisable strategy, except for complaining about the government inadequacy, the League seemed to have partly lost its influence and appeal.

6 Conclusion

Understanding whether the COVID-19 pandemic has damaged or rather benefited populists in Italy is not easy. Whilst the League played this game in opposition, the M5S had an essential role in the management of the crisis. Their institutional role entailed a diverse communication strategy for handling the crisis. Whereas the League tried (with difficulties) to adapt its traditional populist claims to the pandemic emergency, the M5S in line with other mainstream parties addressed the crisis by emphasising the institutional role played. Additionally, the media did not offer an easy ground for classic populist rhetoric. The health emergency—meaning the data on contagion rates, deaths and pressure over the system—and the nature of the pandemic did not need any further media logic elements such as negativity and sensationalism. Consequently, populist claims were dampened and eventually marginalised in media coverage.

Indicators of this shift could be voting intentions in the polls and the relevance that populists had in the public debate and political field, before and after the start of the crisis.

Regarding the polls, the results showed that the League decreased its support during this period (from 32% in January to 27% in May), whilst the M5S has managed to keep its consensus almost consistent, approximately 15–16%.[13] Obviously, these results cannot be attributed only to the crisis. Many other intervening factors could have affected it; however, it is a matter of fact that the League in this period has suffered a loss of consent. Regarding the political and public relevance of these parties, the evidence discussed in this chapter showed that the League and the M5S have had different reactions to the crisis. The main populist flagships of the League, such as anti-immigration claims or law and order proposals, have been weakened because of the ubiquity of the COVID-19 issue. Salvini tried to politicise the issue, particularly blaming the EU; however, his agenda-setting power has been much less strong than before the crisis. The M5S also modified its populist discourse, leaving out usual populist topics—such as political corruption, waste of public money or suspicions about science and "*big pharma*"—and focusing, instead, on managing and responding to the crisis.

All in all, this unusual crisis did not strengthen populist parties—at least not in the short run. By contrast, it defused some populist issues in the public opinion and political debate, on which Salvini was used to hold the ownership. This happened also to the M5S, although in a peculiar way: having to face the pandemic has indeed limited the populist stances of the Movement which, in the face of new, crucial institutional responsibilities, adopted more mainstream positions. Although these changes are certainly temporary, they will likely be the new starting point for a reframe of the populist supply and a redefinition of the Italian political balance in the upcoming post-COVID age.

References

Albertazzi, D., Giovannini, A., & Seddone, A. (2018). 'No Regionalism Please, We Are Leghisti!' The Transformation of the Italian Lega Nord Under the Leadership of Matteo Salvini. *Regional & Federal Studies, 28*(5), 645–671.

[13] Source: www.politico.eu/europe-poll-of-polls/italy/.

Albertazzi, D., & McDonnell, D. (2010). The Lega Nord Back in Government. *West European Politics, 33*(6), 1318–1340.

Bobba, G. (2019). Social Media Populism: Features and 'Likeability' of Lega Nord Communication on Facebook. *European Political Science, 18*(1), 11–23.

Bobba, G., & Legnante, G. (2016). Italy: A Breeding Ground for Populist Political Communication. In T. Aalberg, F. Esser, C. Reinemann, J. Strömbäck, & C. de Vreese (Eds.), *Populist Political Communication in Europe* (pp. 222–234). London: Routledge.

D'Alimonte, R. (2019). How the Populists Won in Italy. *Journal of Democracy, 30*(1), 114–127.

Felstiner, W. L. F., Abel, R. L., & Sarat, A. (1980). The Emergence and Transformation of Disputes: Naming, Blaming, Claiming… *Law & Society Review, 15*(3/4), 631–654.

Mazzoleni, G., & Bracciale, R. (2018). Socially Mediated Populism: The Communicative Strategies of Political Leaders on Facebook. *Palgrave Communications, 4*(1), 1–10.

Mudde, C., & Rovira Kaltwasser, C. (2017). *Populism: A Very Short Introduction.* Oxford and New York: Oxford University Press.

Roncarolo, F., & Cremonesi, C. (2019). Journalistic Narratives and Political Communication Strategies Against the Background of a Critical Mood. In L. Ceccarini & J. L. Newell (Eds.), *The Italian General Election of 2018* (pp. 191–215). Basingstoke: Palgrave Macmillan.

Tarchi, M. (2015). Italy: The Promised Land of Populism? *Contemporary Italian Politics, 7*(3), 273–285.

Tronconi, F. (Ed.). (2015). *Beppe Grillo's Five Star Movement: Organisation, Communication and Ideology.* Farnham: Ashgate.

CHAPTER 5

France: Governmental Unpreparedness as a Discursive Opportunity for Populists

Martin Baloge and Nicolas Hubé

1 Introduction

The handling of the pandemic crisis in France followed the same road as in Italy, although one week later. The identification of the outbreak at the end of February 2020 was unexpected and COVID-19 was seen as a 'Chinese problem' that could not pose a problem for so well-prepared a health system as that in France. This was a mistake and the serious nature of the approaching emergency was for a long time understated as little more than '24-hour flu'. During the first months of 2020, meanwhile, French politics was focused on pension reforms (with massive demonstrations) and on the upcoming local elections (planned for 15 and 22 March). On the policy side, the French health system was not prepared for the shock (not enough face masks, respirators or emergency beds in hospitals) and government communication was erratic, asking people not

M. Baloge · N. Hubé (✉)
Centre for Research on Mediations (CREM),
University of Lorraine, Metz, France
e-mail: nicolas.hube@univ-lorraine.fr

G. Bobba and N. Hubé (eds.), *Populism and the Politicization of the COVID-19 Crisis in Europe*,
https://doi.org/10.1007/978-3-030-66011-6_5

to wear face masks systematically and then saying the opposite a few days later. The political parties had to redefine their strategies and this chapter investigates the diverse roles played during the first four months of the emergency by the two most prominent populist parties, the National Rally (*Rassemblement national*—RN) and Indomitable France (*La France Insoumise*—LFI), whose strategies were hindered by the 'national unity' message. Both parties mixed different strategies, often based on evidence of the lack of medical equipment on the part of the French government.

2 Political Context

France is often mentioned as an early breeding ground for populism. The RN (previously *Front National*—FN) is the 'prototypical populist radical right party' (Mudde and Rovira Kaltwasser 2017: 34) and the oldest institutionalized far-right party in Europe. The new left-populist LFI, meanwhile, was created during the 'new momentum to left-wing populism' in the wake of the euro crisis (ibid.: 37). Over the past decade, both parties have contributed to the general changes in the French party system, in which anti-elitism and media criticism have been used by all political competitors, from the 2007 presidency of Nicolas Sarkozy to the current French President Emmanuel Macron (Cole 2019; Gougou and Persico 2017).

Both played their part in the 'electoral earthquake' (Cole 2019) of the last presidential elections, as four parties took 84.9% of the votes between them in the first round. Macron ended up with 24.01%, 2.7% ahead of Marine Le Pen on 21.3%. The difference between her second place and the fourth position of Jean-Luc Mélenchon (19.6%) was only 618 540 votes, out of a total of 31,381,603 French voters. Conservative François Fillon ended up in third position with 20.01%. Due to the electoral system in France, their results were not so good one month later at the general elections (see Table 1). The RN/FN and LFI have not always had the same electoral success. After Jean-Marie Le Pen's qualification for the second round of the Presidential election in 2002 (16.9%), the party came in fourth in 2007 (10.4%), losing voters to Nicolas Sarkozy, and the decade that followed was not a successful one. However, since the 2012 Presidential election (17.9%, third position), the party has maintained its votes at a high level, coming first in the 2015 regional and 2019 European elections. Here lies the main difference with LFI, whose sole success (for the moment) was the latest Presidential election, before losing more than 5.6 million voters within two years, between 2017 and 2019.

Table 1 Main French political parties (>5% in the last general election)

Political party	*2017 general election*		*2019 European election*	
	Vote shares	*Seats*	*Vote shares*	*Seats*
In power				
La République en Marche (The Republic on the Move)	43.1	306	22.4	23
Modem	6.1	42		
Union des Démocrates et Indépendants	3	17		
In opposition				
La France Insoumise (Indomitable France)	4.9	17	6.3	6
Parti Socialiste (Socialist Party)	5.7	30	6.2	6
Les Verts (Greens)	0.1	1	13.5	13
Les Républicains (The Republicans)	22.2	112	8.5	8
Rassemblement National (National Rally)/Front National	8.8	8	23.3	23

The FN (now RN) has typical far-right roots in the anti-Semitic, anti-communist, xenophobic, ultra-conservative and/or fascist traditions, but has succeeded in moving 'from pariah to republican democratic contender' (Mondon 2014). In 2011, in preparation for the 2012 elections, Jean-Marie Le Pen (83 years old) gave way to his second daughter Marine. With the help of young public relations staff and technocrats, she succeeded in framing her arrival as the sign of the party's 'normalisation' and 'respectability', despite being from the hard wing of the party. Following the same 'de-demonisation' approach, the party changed its name in 2018 and became the RN. Due to the peculiarities of the French electoral system, the party has few elected members: in 2019, 20 MEPs, 6 MPs, 1 Senator; and, since the end of June 2020, 10 mayors (but only 1 in a city with more than 100,000 inhabitants) and 5 additional mayors who are close to the party without officially representing it.

The story of Mélenchon and his party is very different, having started on the left wing of the mainstream Socialist Party (PS). After the 2002 defeat against Le Pen, his view was that the party should become more leftist. After the second presidential defeat in 2007, he left the PS in 2008 along with other socialists to found a new left-wing party, inspired by the German example of Oscar Lafontaine's Die Linke in 2007.

This small party made an alliance with the Communist Party and another small party to form the Left Front coalition, under the banner of which Mélenchon took part in the Presidential elections in 2012, and in the 2009 and 2014 European Parliament elections. After 2012, he radicalized his message with more provocative populist tones, inspired by Podemos, Syriza and Bernie Sanders (Castaño 2018). In 2016, LFI was created as an eco-socialist movement, an electoral machine based on a horizontal hierarchy. It is a movement and not a party. In 2019, the party had 17 MPs, 2 Senators and 5 MEPs.

3 COVID-19 Diffusion and Political Measures

During the *first phase* of COVID-19, the pandemic was framed as a foreign disease. After warnings from the World Health Organization and the European Centre for Disease Prevention and Control, France did not take specific measures, although the country did have some very early cases. Five days after the first official deaths in China, a Chinese tourist in Paris was diagnosed on 16 January and died one month later. Eight days later, three French people returning from China were also diagnosed. On 30 January, a plane brought 200 French people back from Wuhan and they were placed in isolation. During this phase, the whole political sphere was focused on the upcoming local elections that were scheduled to take place on 15 and 22 March (and also on pensions reform). The Minister for Health even took the liberty of resigning on 16 February to stand in as her party's candidate for the upcoming municipal election for the Paris mayor's office, as the previous candidate was caught up in a sex-tape scandal.

The situation suddenly changed at the end of February with the first death of a French person (26 February) (Fig. 1 and Table 2). The government announced the *second phase* two days after, with bans on large groups meeting. The perception of the danger of the pandemic changed with the lockdown measures in Italy and the increasing number of infections and deaths. One week later, the government announced a 'reinforced step 2': closing of schools in two departments, requisitioning of the stock of face masks, fixing the price of disinfectant gels, and, more symbolically, the closing of the annual agricultural fair, always a political highlight and especially so just two weeks before elections. During that week, President Macron consulted the Presidents of the two Chambers of Parliament, those of the political groups and decided to go ahead with the

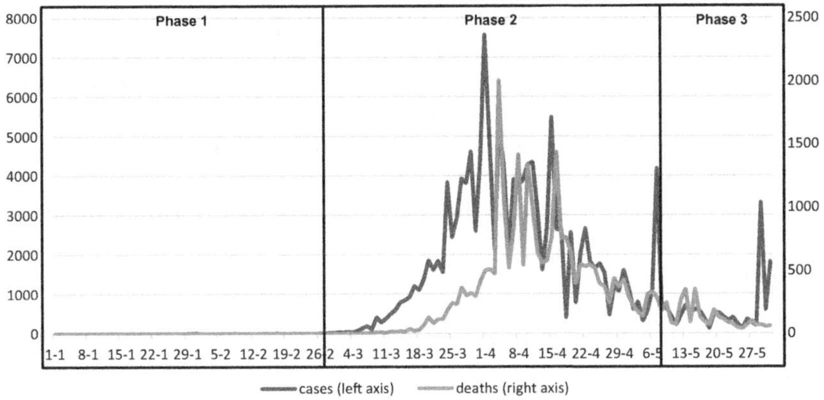

Fig. 1 Daily death toll and new cases in France (*Source* European Centre for Disease Prevention and Control. Phase 1: pre-COVID-19; Phase 2: spread and containment measures; Phase 3: contagion mitigation)

Table 2 COVID-19 pandemic in France

Cases	154,591
Total deaths	29,296
Total recovered	71,506
Cases for 1 M pop	2369
Deaths for 1 M pop	449

Source www.worldometers.info/coronavirus/ (update 10/6/2020)

elections, arguing that the scientific committee was not against it. On 12 March, Macron made the first of a series of TV addresses. The whole educational system (from kindergarten to university) was to be closed on 16 March, one day after the first round of elections. Two days later, Prime Minister Philippe announced that France had reached *phase 3* of the pandemic with a strict lockdown. The day after the elections, Macron gave his second TV address, justifying the closure of the borders, the restriction of public liberties, and preparing public opinion for a longer period of lockdown. In his third TV address (24 March), in a live broadcast from a field hospital, he presented the pandemic as a 'war' and launched a military operation to ease pressure on the overloaded hospitals in the East of France. Every day, a ministerial press conference was broadcast live in the different media, giving the latest update on the pandemic situation. President Macron then stopped his TV addresses, appearing again only at the end of March in Angers to announce a new delivery of masks and (with the same warlike rhetoric) to launch a new 'national sovereignty' approach to health-policy. He appeared again on 13 April to announce the extension of the lockdown until 11 May. What would happen in *phase 3* was then explained one week later by the Prime Minister during a two-hour press conference.

Phase 3 started slowly after 11 May: some regions remained half-closed, but schools could start to open some classes (but not all and not the universities), freedom of movement remained limited to a 100 km radius, while access to bars and restaurants was also restricted. The second round of the local election was to be held on 28 June. President Macron then accelerated the transition on 14 June, announcing that schools must be open from 21 June until 5 July, when the summer vacations started. Most of the restriction measures were lifted, and the last restrictions on public liberties (mainly border controls) were removed on 9 July. The results of the local elections on 28 June were a disaster for Macron's party. Apart from the re-election of the Prime Minister in his own town, they did not succeed in winning any cities. In Paris, Macron's candidate came in third position.

4 Populist Discourse at the Time of COVID-19

The emergence of the pandemic in France transformed some aspects of the messages put across by the leaders of the RN and LFI. The COVID crisis came in the aftermath of a very dense period politically, characterized by weeks of demonstrations against the pension reform proposed by President Macron and by the campaign for the municipal elections held on the eve of the lockdown. The first few weeks of the year were therefore mainly devoted to pension reform, leading Mélenchon to publish Facebook posts such as '*Pension reform is only in the interest of the employers of financial companies. The productive employers of this country must say y a basta to the financial employers. Because it is the productive bosses who are paying for the financial bosses*' (30/01/2020) or Le Pen '*The government is setting France ablaze with a pension reform that is challenging a system to which the French were attached, and which will cost 5 to 10 times more than the deficit it was supposed to cover…. I demand a REFERENDUM!*' (14/01/2020). Each leader was thus true to the ideological line of their party and condemned the national elites, especially Macron. Le Pen focused on issues of insecurity and immigration ('*I am afraid that Emmanuel Macron is only interested in the issue of Islamist communitarianism for electoral reasons. In reality, unfortunately, he doesn't care about all this, he doesn't understand where the problem lies*', Le Pen's Facebook page 26/02/2020) while Mélenchon, for example, focused on the issue of fundamental rights and freedoms ('*Macron gives the police the right to censor websites*', Mélenchon's Facebook page, 23/01/2020). The classic dimensions of populism were at work here, with criticism of the elites (also journalists, referred to by Mélenchon as '*the media of the officialdom*'), defence of the people (e.g., by calling for a referendum in the case of Le Pen or the Popular Initiative Referendum in the case of Mélenchon) and opposition to 'others' in the case of the president of the RN, mainly meaning migrants. Until the week before the lockdown, only five Facebook posts out of 404 were dedicated to the COVID-19 crisis. On France and China, Le Pen surprisingly posted on 29 January: '*Nothing, absolutely nothing, justifies our compatriots of Chinese origin being victims of mistrust because of the coronavirus. They have nothing to do with it after all! Let us remain intelligent and fraternal!*'. Interestingly, the pandemic was denounced as nothing more than a strategic pitch to force through pension reform (Le Pen's Facebook page, 29/02/2020).

The change came during the lockdown, as the period of elections and demonstrations was totally overshadowed by the COVID-19 crisis. The old themes were dropped on the whole, as the political news became entirely focused, for weeks on end, on the management and effects of this crisis. Pension reform was even postponed by the President of the Republic. However, the populist rhetoric was not abandoned, merely transposed to this new and unprecedented issue. The people were still held up as the absolute reference, as when Le Pen maintained that '*The people have the right to the TRUTH*' on the subject of mask policy or Mélenchon stated that decisions on health matters should be taken in such a way that '*the people are the only ones to ensure common salvation in complete independence*' (13 April 2020). Criticism of the elites also continued, sometimes in very vague terms for the president of the LFI ('*Ladies and gentlemen the powerful*', 13/04/2020) or more directly targeted against the government (as when Le Pen wrote: '*Three months of government LIES: I invite you to share this video massively!*', 7/04/2020). The main difference between the two, if we focus on the attributes of populism, was that Le Pen was the only one targeting social groups seen as not part of the people, even in times of health crisis. The President of the RN thus pitted French senior citizens against immigrants, claiming that the latter being given preference in the management of mask stocks, as she declared on 15 April that '*Masks for migrant centres and not for our retirement homes? Join me in denouncing this absolute SCANDAL!*'

The COVID-19 crisis did not fundamentally change the communication styles of the two leaders. Criticism of the elites (mainly the government and the presidency) remained strong, while references to the people did not weaken. This was partly due to the fact that the two leaders continued to be invited regularly by the media during the lockdown period. The crisis thus provided them with another opportunity to mobilize people in favour of (or against) more or less clearly identified groups: healthcare workers and the French, but also public services, as when Mélenchon declared that '*everywhere the epidemic will encounter health systems that are already largely under strain due to policies to reduce spending on public services*' (10/03/2020).

Hindered by the discourse of national unity that could make their criticism seem indecent, the two MPs used the most legitimate political tool at their disposal: their legislative activities in a time of semi-lockdown in parliament. Mélenchon asked the government two written questions and Le Pen five about the management of the pandemic. She also submitted three oral questions to the Government on this subject. However, it is interesting to note that in the National Assembly, both elected representatives linked this issue with their traditional ideological concerns. Le Pen thus linked COVID with immigration: '*Madam Secretary of State, Minister, my question is simple: on 10 August 1932, a law was passed to protect the national workforce during the Great Depression after the 1929 crisis; do you intend to present, in the same spirit, a text in order to abolish postings of workers from abroad, to establish national priority and thus respond to the social crisis resulting from the health crisis?*' (Facebook page, 18/05/2020). Mélenchon, meanwhile, focused on social matters by asking the government '*that an unconditional and equal bonus be announced for all health sector personnel. Furthermore, he […] asks whether the salaries of these professionals, who have given so much, will be increased*' (Facebook page, 2/06/2020).

5 The Politicization of COVID-19 Issue by Populists

The COVID crisis was highly politicized by both parties. For both organizations, this politicization consisted in presenting the pandemic as a manifestation of the shortcomings of Macron's presidency. It is worth noting that the trilogy of 'naming, blaming, claiming' (Felstiner et al. 1980) was not followed through the phases of the crisis. Before phase 2, both populist leaders were silent and after that, they were permanently switching from one argument to another. However, as we have seen in the previous section, the two leaders handled this politicization in different ways.

Looking at their Facebook communication (until 31 May), Mélenchon was much more engaged in *naming* the problems than Le Pen (41.4% versus 30.2%), while the RN leader was *blaming* the government more frequently (37.1%) than her LFI opponent (18.9): 'Government lies and unpreparedness' (21/03/2020) was the motto of her communication during the whole period. Both used *claiming* in similar proportions, in one in every four posts (25.2% for Mélenchon and 24.1% for Le Pen). These strategies emerged spectacularly from week 12 onwards. At this point, when lockdown was becoming a reality for the French, the two leaders began an enterprise of politicizing and highlighting (*naming*, 14 posts) this issue and, at the same time, in similar proportions, *blaming* the government for its *unpreparedness* (9 posts) and *claiming* quick answers (8 posts), during this week. In comparison, two weeks earlier, in week 10, there was only one *naming* post and none using *blaming* or *claiming*, although the news was already partly focused on the spread of COVID-19. Everything was therefore happening as if the lockdown had acted like a match, setting fire to the debates, offering the two leaders a clear opportunity to take ownership of the subject, mainly by criticizing the government and the presidency. Weeks 13–16 were thus marked by a very intense period (but never as intense as in week 12) when the two leaders posted messages on Facebook based on *naming*, *blaming* and *claiming*.

The main arguments put forward by the two leaders with regard to *blaming* were based on the health management issues of the crisis. Mélenchon thus used both *naming* and *blaming* strategies when he wrote on 20 May 2020: '*Another Macron lie about masks: I had warned about this issue as early as the beginning of February... The French have the right to the TRUTH*'. He had also posted two days before: '*How can the President dare to say this when his government has LIED about the very usefulness of masks precisely to hide the shortage? These remarks are an unbearable provocation given the situation!*' (18/05/2020). The masks issue, as well as that of tests, was indeed the main topic at stake for the whole political sphere. Le Pen, who also condemned the Government's action on this issue ('*Today I was the guest of France 3 [a public media channel] to speak about easing the lockdown, the URGENT and IMPERATIVE supply of masks to the population and the shortcomings of the government and its bureaucracy in managing this crisis*', 19/04/2020), also used claiming strategies by writing: '*We voted in the Assembly for 5.5% VAT on masks. Why aren't we seeing this cut in prices in stores?! The same goes for sanitizer gel…*' (5/05/2020). However, the controversy was not only focused on health issues. Indeed, it revealed the difficulties being encountered by the French public hospitals system. The images broadcast on social networks of healthcare workers forced to protect themselves with garbage bags found an echo with the indignant leader of LFI: 'Caregivers are forced to use rubbish bags because they don't have gowns provided by the State. Unworthy of the world's 6th largest economy. We will not forget those responsible for such a disgrace to our public services. It is their policy that should be thrown away' (8/04/2020). Returning to his left-wing ideology, the health issue then also became an economic, budget, fiscal and ideological issue. '*What should be done about the debt?*' asked Mélenchon in the midst of this crisis.

More generally, this period was characterized by different public health controversies giving rise to blaming. Some were caused directly by the government: one week after the first round of the elections, previous Health Minister Agnès Buzyn acknowledged in an interview that, when she had resigned, she was '*crying because I was aware of the tsunami that was ahead of us…*'. Both leaders reacted directly, pointing to this mismanagement as an affair of State: '*If Agnes Buzyn's statements reflect the truth, this is a very serious scandal for the State. Ms. Buzyn will probably have to explain herself to the Court of Justice, perhaps the High Court will have to be seized…*' (Le Pen). In a long message, Mélenchon described Agnes Buzyn's confession as '*appalling […] Did she know and warn people three months in advance? And if so, why wasn't anything done? Why is she telling this story now when it's too late? Does she realize that she is criminally responsible for herself and for others, people she claims to have warned?*'. In the meantime, 90 legal proceedings have been initiated. The

National Assembly and Senate have also opened parliamentary inquiries (respectively, on 26 May and 30 June).

In the face of these critics, the government tried to depoliticize the situation. In an unprecedented move, Prime Minister, Edouard Philippe, and Health Minister, Olivier Véran, organized a press conference on March 18 in the presence of three scientists: Professor Jérôme Salomon, Director General of Health, and Professors Karine Lacombe and Arnaud Fontanet. The tone was deliberately neutral, backed up by graphs and figures in order to depoliticize the political crisis that was beginning to emerge. Mélenchon acknowledged that '*the Prime Minister's information effort is necessary*', while describing the conference as '*less showy than the President's communication*' (Twitter account, 28/03/2020), but the controversies surrounding the masks and other lack of preparedness did not really cease. Macron's communication was accused of denying the facts (Mélenchon's Facebook page, 19/05/2020), as attested by the healthcare officers and the press: '*they're trying to be neither responsible nor guilty*!' (Le Pen's Facebook account, 5/05/2020).

These polemics are of course observed in the media as they are reflected in the official counting of media attendance of these parties in April 2020, in the midst of the pandemics.[1] On the two main TV channels, the presidential party and the executive have had the most air time (527 min), followed by the Republicans (144.19), LFI (70.16), the PS (69.03), the RN (54.03) and the Green Party (33.27). On the news channels, the populist parties are quite far behind the traditional parties. During the month of April, Le Pen was invited once on one of the main national radio station, Mélenchon on no occasion.

French public debate also focused on the chloroquine (HCQ) issue from the early days of phase 2, when epidemiologist Professor Didier Raoult announced on YouTube that his experiment would solve the problem. In true populist style, he denounced the pharmaceutical companies, criticized all his opponents and polarized the debate. During the peak of the crisis (22 March–9 April), he was supported by the mainstream conservative opposition (Les Républicains) and Macron himself visited him in the first days of April. At the end of May, HCQ was forbidden to cure COVID-19. The two leaders also sought to be seen as close to the scientist. On 26 March, Mélenchon gave the broad outlines

[1] https://www.csa.fr/csapluralisme/tableau. (Last consulted in November 2020).

of a telephone conversation he had had with Professor Raoult, praising '*the calm, courtesy and smiling tone*' of the scientist and pointing out that '*Didier Raoult is too unpopular among the beautiful people not to arouse interest. Especially when it comes from friends of Madame Buzyn [former Minister of Health]. The woman who knew and lied*'. The scientific controversy therefore fuelled political controversy as well. Le Pen also sought to present herself as an advocate of Didier Raoult, speaking out on 22 March to laud '*The generalization of clinical trials for the chloroquine and azithromycin-based treatment of Professor Didier Raoult, announced by Health Minister Olivier Véran, is good news. FINALLY! Let's not close any option when facing the coronavirus!*'.

The entire crisis period was therefore subject to intense controversy and considerable politicization of health issues, from several angles: scientific, political, budget, moral, etc. The RN differentiated itself from Mélenchon by *claiming* a closure of all borders. Mélenchon, meanwhile, tried not to present only short-term policy answers. On 13 April, he presented LFI as an alternative for government: '*We can rule differently with other goals and methods. And we are willing to claim that we can start to do so at any time. That is why our contribution is a programme for government*', setting out different measures.

6 Conclusion

The COVID crisis has not been without its political effects in France. The parties described as populist have both been heavily involved in this issue, focusing their criticism on the government and Macron himself. In particular, Le Pen made extensive use of the strategy of blaming political actors, while Mélenchon opted more for the strategy of naming these issues as broader political ones. After being an issue of secondary importance (coming after pension reform and the local elections), in both cases, the turning point came at the moment of the lockdown when the subject became unavoidable and monopolized the speeches of the two leaders.

This strategy does not seem to have really moved the lines, however, or gained popular support for either party. On the one hand, opinion polls show that voting intentions for the 2022 presidential elections have not moved[2]: Le Pen even lost one percentage point over the whole

[2] Source: https://www.politico.eu/europe-poll-of-polls/france/. (Last consulted in November 2020).

period, while Mélenchon and Macron remained stable. On the other hand, the municipal elections of June 2020 were a failure overall for all three parties (RN, LFI and LREM). The RN thus won only one municipality of more than 100,000 inhabitants (Perpignan) and now has only 840 council seats in 258 municipalities, against 1438 seats in 463 municipalities in 2014, and lost some municipalities (one district of Marseille, for example). For this election, LFI chose not to form an autonomous list and decided instead to participate in left-wing citizen's lists, but this 'choice did not work', according to Mélenchon. Macron's party was also severely defeated, only managing to win two cities of significant size: Le Havre (through Prime Minister Edouard Philippe) and Amiens (where Macron comes from). Ultimately, the health crisis and exhaustion of the French party system seem to have mainly benefited the traditional mainstream parties of government (LR and the PS, with the latter putting an end to its string of defeats by keeping control of Paris and Lille, for example) and the Ecologists, who managed to win by joining forces with other left-wing parties (PS) in large cities such as Marseille, Bordeaux, Strasbourg, Lyon, Grenoble or Montpellier. But these elections were also marked by a very high abstention rate (58% in the second round). Although the populist strategy did not work in this local election, the state of French democracy still seems fragile today, and while there is nothing to indicate that populist parties will take advantage of this in 2022, everything suggests that the French political game, after this health crisis, has become even more blurred.

References

Castaño, P. (2018). Populisme de gauche en Europe: une comparaison entre Podemos et La France insoumise. *Mouvements, 96*, 169–180.

Cole, A. (2019). *Emmanuel Macron and the Remaking of France*. Manchester: Manchester University Press.

Felstiner, W. L. F., Abel, R. L., & Sarat, A. (1980). The Emergence and Transformation of Disputes: Naming, Blaming, Claiming... *Law & Society Review, 15*(3/4), 631–654.

Gougou, F., & Persico, S. (2017). A New Party System in the Making? The 2017 French Presidential Election. *French Politics, 15*, 303–321.

Mondon, A. (2014). The Front National in the Twenty-First Century: From Pariah to Republican Democratic Contender? *Modern & Contemporary France, 22*(3), 301–320.

Mudde, C., & Rovira Kaltwasser, C. (2017). *Populism: A Very Short Introduction*. Oxford and New York: Oxford University Press.

CHAPTER 6

Germany: The AfD's Staggering Between Reason and Resistance

Oliver W. Lembcke

1 Introduction

As the first right-wing party entering Parliament at the federal level, the AfD's aim is to challenge the established parties and to signify a rupture of German politics in style and action. The COVID-19 crisis could have been another boost for the AfD, considering the fact that the party has only grown bigger in times of crisis: It emerged from the financial crisis and the widespread critique of the EZB's EURO policy. Furthermore, the AfD had a streak of successful elections in the wake of the migration crisis in Germany. However, the AfD does not look like a profiteer from this pandemic, and this chapter tries to explain why. This chapter argues that struggles between the governments at the federal level ('Bund') and at the state level ('Länder') have absorbed most of the media attention during the early stages of the pandemic, which made it rather difficult for the AfD to get its own message out. Moreover, the AfD has been limiting

O. W. Lembcke (✉)
Ruhr-University Bochum, Bochum, Germany
e-mail: oliver.lembcke@ruhr-uni-bochum.de

G. Bobba and N. Hubé (eds.), *Populism and the Politicization of the COVID-19 Crisis in Europe*,
https://doi.org/10.1007/978-3-030-66011-6_6

its critique to highlighting the government's failures in prevention and to stressing mistakes made in effectively managing the crisis. Consequently, the AfD could not exert the same radical critique (in style and content) as for example during the migration crisis. Nevertheless, the AfD has refused to participate in the overall COVID-19 consensus by politicizing the issue. Finally, it also tried to radicalize its critique by switching from a 'safety first' strategy to a strategy of 'individual rights first'. Nevertheless, it seems that the party has been suffering from some 'outbidding' by forms of extra-parliamentary opposition (APO), which oppose the government's COVID-19 policies and are much more resistant, radical, and in some ways also more populist than the AfD itself.

2 Political Context

The result of the 2017 federal elections has had a decisive impact on the political situation in Germany. On the one hand, the governing coalition of CDU, Bavarian CSU and SPD has succeeded in renewing its alliance. On the other hand, the great coalition between the Christian Democrats and the Social Democrats is also the coalition of the biggest losers of this election. As a result, the government does have relatively secure parliamentary majorities, and its room for manoeuvre is de facto limited due to internal tensions (especially within the SPD). From the beginning, the breakup of the coalition hovered over Merkel's fourth cabinet like a sword of Damocles.

The difficulty in forming a stable government at the federal level did not come as a surprise. The election trend at the state level clearly shows that government coalitions in Germany are increasingly based on mathematical majorities, but no longer on ideological agreement between the coalition partners. One of the key factors for this development is the end of the two-party dominance. The CDU's future as a catch-all party is unclear; that of the SPD is already history due to lack of voter approval. While both parties were able to retain over 80% of votes well into the 1980s, nowadays the voter's support is only just over 50% (see Table 1).

In the wake of these erosion processes, the fragmentation and polarization of the German party system have been growing since the reunification of Germany—a trend that forms the ideal breeding ground for the emergence of new parties, especially on the fringes of the party system. Based on the Laakso-Taagepera index (Laakso and Taagepera

Table 1 Main German political parties (>5% in the last general election)

Political party	*General Election 2017*		*2019 European election*	
	Vote shares (%)	*Seats*	*Vote shares (%)*	*Seats*
In power				
Christian Democrats (CDU)	26.9	200	22.6	23
Christian Democrats in Bavaria (CSU)	6.2	46	6.3	6
Social Democrats (SPD)	20.5	153	15.8	16
In opposition				
Right-Wing Populists (AfD)	12.6	94	11.0	11
Liberals (FDP)	10.7	80	5.4	5
Socialists (Left Party)	9.2	69	5.5	5
Greens (B 90/Die Grünen)	8.9	67	20.5	21

1979), the German party system at the federal level is now more fragmented than it was in 1949. The governing parties are reacting to this situation by redefining their programs and changing personnel, but in both cases without much success. Both governing parties currently have no centre of power, which further damages the government's ability to act. One exception to this is the Bavarian regional party CSU, which, after its poor performance in 2017, has succeeded in repositioning itself under the leadership of Minister President Söder.

The main beneficiaries of the government's weakness have been the right-wing populists of the AfD and, after a disappointing result in the 2017 election, the Greens. On the contrary, the Socialists and the Liberals have so far been unable to benefit in a similar fashion. The successes of the Greens and the AfD reflect not least an East-West divide, which is also of European relevance (Ignazi 1992), as the recent European elections have shown: The West is becoming 'greener' with 'green, alternative and liberal' (GAL) values, while the East is becoming 'bluer' favouring 'traditional, authoritarian and national' (TAN) positions. This is particularly true in Germany, the once divided country. When the AfD was founded in 2011, it was a Western 'professor's party' under the leadership of Lucke, rallying against the monetary policy of the EU and against the euro. Thereafter the focus shifted more to an Eastern political style under Petry. With this shift in the party's base, the ideological core has changed to become more defined by TAN positions (Rosenfelder 2017).

In the Eastern German states, the AfD has now established itself as a strong, if not the strongest, opposition party; in the West, however, it still has the character of a fringe party, although it is much more strongly represented in the Southwest than in the northern city states of Hamburg and Bremen or in the most populous state of North Rhine-Westphalia (Manow 2018). For the moment, the AfD has no real chance of participating in West-German governments. This was demonstrated not least by the Thuringian elections in 2019, in which the liberal candidate was surprisingly elected Minister President with the votes of the CDU and AfD, but had to resign after a few days because of the general public's outrage that he has been put into office with the help of right-wing populists. No power in the sense of 'coalition potential' (Sartori 1976) can be ascribed to the AfD. However, it has 'blackmail potential' since the party has issue-ownership in the policy field of migration and can put pressure on right of the centre parties. Moreover, the AfD has considerable influence on the arithmetic of government formation.

3 COVID-19 Diffusion and Political Measures

The measures of the German Federal Government and the state governments to contain the spread of COVID-19 in Germany can be divided into three phases (pre-COVID-19, spread and containment measures, and contagion mitigation). In view of the fact that the outbreak of COVID-19 in China was officially detected already on December 1, 2019, the pre-COVID-19 phase in Germany lasted quite long. On February 26, 2020, the government revaluated the severity of the situation: Previously, there had been isolated cases of infected persons in Germany, but at that point, according to the BMG, it was no longer possible to trace the spread of the infection due to missing links in the infection chain (Fig. 1 and Table 2).

The changed assessment of the situation resulted in a tightening of measures implemented to contain the pandemic. While the federal government initially limited itself to measures to educate and inform the population, advising to take hygienic precautions (disinfection, hand washing) and to keep distance (social distancing); the second phase saw a relatively rapid transition to regulatory intervention supported by the media that seemed to share to a large extent the government's assessments. The direct measures to contain COVID-19 were still orchestrated quite uniformly at the beginning of the second phase by the German government with the support of the RKI. The RKI defined limit values

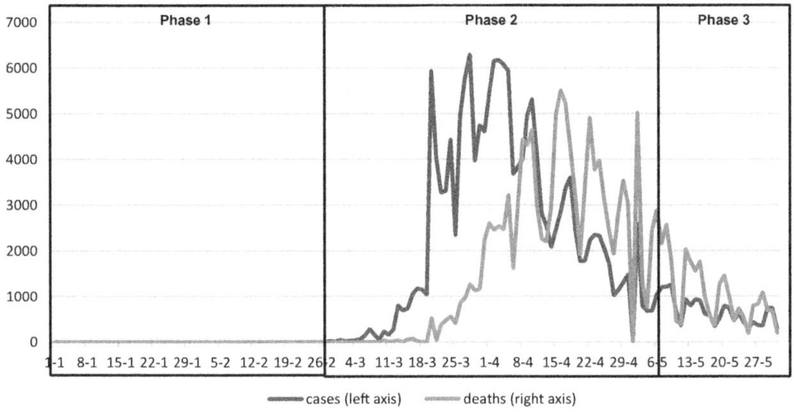

Fig. 1 Daily death toll and new cases in Germany (*Source* European Center for Disease Prevention and Control. Phase 1: pre-COVID-19; Phase 2: spread and containment measures; Phase 3: contagion mitigation)

Table 2 COVID-19 pandemic in Germany

Cases	186,525
Total deaths	8831
Total recovered	170,700
Cases for 1 M pop	2227
Deaths for 1 M pop	105

Source www.worldometers.info/Coronavirus/ (update 10/6/2020)

and risk areas and made recommendations for the measures to be taken. Soon there was consensus that returnees from risk areas had to undergo a two-week quarantine (starting from April 10, 2020), and social distancing also became a general rule of behaviour in Germany. Soon, however, a Babylonian babble of voices became apparent as a result of the federal division of powers under the German constitution. According to the Constitution, the states and municipalities are responsible for interpreting and implementing the necessary measures. Thus Bavaria, as a neighbour to Austria, became the forerunner of a particularly strict COVID-19 policy that other federal states did not want to follow. And the general obligation to wear a mask was first introduced by the city of Jena on April 6, 2020, despite the fact that the infection figures in the whole of Thuringia, were well below the federal average.

However, the regulations were not limited to the acute danger of infection but extended to the entire economic and cultural life in Germany, bringing it to a 'lockdown' (March 16, 2020). Not only were mass events, such as the soccer league or music concerts cancelled, but all public institutions were closed to visitors, including schools, kindergartens and universities. Cultural places, bars or restaurants were closed. Only 'systemically relevant' activities remained accessible, including grocery stores, especially supermarkets, and, in some places, drugstores and home improvement stores. All retail sales were prohibited unless the very restrictive safety regulations for employees were guaranteed. Companies switched to short-time work or to home office. These regulations were accompanied by various forms of government economic aid. For example, the short-time work allowance was reintroduced, which had already helped to alleviate the problem of unemployment during the financial crisis of 2008/2009. In addition, emergency aid measures were offered for the first three months to cover *operating* expenses (e.g. office rent). The fact that this did not include the real cost of living has brought criticism of the federal government and the state governments involved, which, however, did not resonate too much in the media.

The third phase resulting in a relaxation of the restrictive measures started in Germany on May 6, 2020. The German government and the state governments agreed on common standards for infection control. According to these standards, counties and cities are only obliged to reinstate COVID-19 measures if more than 50 new infections per 100,000 inhabitants can be detected within seven days. The obligation to wear a mask and to socially distance remain in force. Under these conditions, not only companies and stores can reopen, but also public institutions, provided that the organizers can present an appropriate hygiene concept. This has contributed to a considerable normalization of life, allowing schools and kindergartens to reopen. In addition, cultural and sporting events are allowed to take place again, provided that government guidelines can be upheld.

In addition to the regulatory measures, government action was also characterized by several structural measures aimed at protecting the healthcare system from possible overburdening by COVID-19 patients. By the end of the first phase, the BMG had already initiated the massive purchase of personal protective clothing (PPE), particularly masks. At the beginning of the second phase, government regulations and initiatives were intended to increase the supply resources in hospitals, with a particular focus on the capacity of intensive care beds (ICB). As a result, these capacities were never exhausted in Germany at any time (the percentage of free ICB was never less than 34% during the time from April 16 to June 30). On the contrary, individual German states have made their resources available for the reception of COVID-19 patients from France and Italy. For some time now, however, the question has been investigated, initiated by some media reports, whether the government's subsidies have led to false incentives and deadweight effects.

Despite the fact that the health care system has passed the acid test for the time being, the pandemic has resulted in a considerable slump of the German economy. Forecasts unanimously expect considerable growth in 2021. However, it is highly questionable whether it will be able to compensate for the decrease of more than 6% in 2020. The same is applicable to the medium-term effects of the COVID-19 crisis on the German economy, which is still heavily dependent on exports. Indeed, there are clear signs of job loss and a shrinking of future opportunities for Generation Z, which is likely to be only marginally prepared for this challenged economy.

4 Populist Discourse at the Time of COVID-19

It is commonplace that times of crisis favour the government. It is able to act while the opposition can only stand by and watch. In such situations, consensus-oriented cooperation often imposes itself as an opposition strategy to prove that the government is aware of its responsibilities. All parties, except for the AfD, adopted such an attitude during the COVD-19 crisis. For the AfD, the pandemic is proof of the incapacity of the country's elites. According to the AfD, the government's incapacity has three reasons (Stefan Keuter, 07/05/2020).[1]

First, the government under Merkel's leadership has not been able to recognize the challenge of the pandemic in time (e.g. Weidel, 04/03/2020), although the Coronavirus has long been acknowledged as a pandemic threat (Kraft, 12/02/2020). Secondly, it has failed to take precautions for emergencies, and instead, with its eyes wide open, has foolishly relied on foreign countries (e.g. Spangenberg, 12/02/2020), in

[1] All mentions in Sects. 4 and 5 are coming from the Bundestag debates ('Plenarprotokolle'). Due to place limitation, the references only give names and date.

particular China (Keinwächter, 13/03/2020) and the WHO (Oehme, 28/05/2020). Thirdly, the government's crisis management lacks any sense of proportion, because it presents the lockdown as the only possible solution (Komning, 14/05/2020), but ignores the harsh consequences for the people (Keuter, 07/05/2020) and the economy (Hilse, 18/06/2020).

Although there are voices within the AfD calling for constructive cooperation in view of the crisis (Pohl, 25/03/2020)—even from prominent figures such as Alice Weidel (04/03/2020), the co-chair of the AfD parliamentary group in the German Bundestag—they remain isolated. Instead, they portray themselves as the only 'alternative' to the pandemic consensus of the other parties and as a true oppositional force for whom the topic of COVID-19 is not only a top priority (Robby Schlund, 12/02/2020), but who also fights to ensure that families are heard as the real sufferers of the pandemic (Reichardt, 22/04/2020). This issue has been hammered away since March (e.g. Kleinwächter, 28/05/2020). The AfD is now demanding unrestricted solidarity for families, financially (Pohl, 25/03/2020) and organizationally, i.e. by reopening schools and kindergartens as soon as possible (Schlund, 22/04/2020).

Moreover, the family support is also used as a cipher for taking care of the people—the German people (Hampel, 11/03/2020). Accordingly, in the international race for the vaccine, it is essential to protect the German people (Gauland, 25/03/2020), always according to the motto: 'Germany first, Germany first' (Müller, 23/4/2020). For the crisis now reveals what the other parties could not see or admit (Harald Weyel, 23/4/2020), namely that only the nation state has the necessary capacity to act, but not the EU. European cooperation can complement national politics, but it cannot replace it, because it is unable to represent German interests (Gauland, 25/03/2020). In the opinion of the AfD, it is simply not in Germany's interest to see the pandemic as an opportunity for European solidarity, let alone for deepening the European economic and financial integration via 'Corona bonds' (Boehringer, 25/03/2020). Even the admission of intensive care patients from neighbouring countries, which has been understood and endorsed by many in public discourse as a symbolic gesture, must be kept within limits according to the AfD (Spangenberg, 07/05/2020).

In the AfD's opinion, the inability of the other parties to draw boundaries is one of the fundamental evils of German politics, which has been particularly evident in migration policy. Now the government is prone to make the same mistakes again: For instance, why are German countrymen not allowed to travel to the German coasts, while refugees are allowed into the country without quarantine (Hemmelgarn, 13/05/2020)? Further, why should Germany pay 'the many billions for the asylum industry', when its public finances will be under considerable strain for the foreseeable future as a result of the COVID-19 crisis? (Jacobi, 25/03/2020). Finally, when will the German government learn the lessons from the migration crisis and invest more in efficient border protection, which also provides the means to protect the German people against an import of COVID-19 (Kleinwächter, 11/03/2020)?

In short, according to the AfD's interpretation, the government is incapable. This is the unanimous verdict within the AfD. And one of the decisive reasons for this, in their view, is that the government cannot think in genuinely political categories: national identity and national interest. Instead, it follows scientific suggestions and tries to hide the fact that its COVID-19 policies, like all political decisions, create 'winners and losers' as a result. The partner in crime is the media. As it has been before, the so-called mainstream media are the real scapegoats in this pandemic, according to the AfD, because they systematically suppress necessary criticism of the government (Reichardt, 07/05/2020) or stigmatize dissenting opinions, especially those of the AfD, portraying them as conspiracy theorists, Corona-deniers, or 'Covidiots' (Komning, 14/05/2020). Occasionally, however, these attacks have been self-inflicted by murmuring coming from the AfD about the Bill and Melinda Gates Foundation and its influence on COVID-19 (e.g. Braun, 15/05/2020).

Against this background, it is obvious that the AfD is seeking to establish a link to the demonstrations against the state's COVID-19 policy that have started in May 2020 immediately in the wake of the loosening of restrictions. The AfD welcomes these events as civil rights protest (e.g. Sichert, 14/05/2020). However, these protests also show very clearly the limited political impact of the AfD during the Corona crisis. For the party is not able to bind or even channel the protests. In fact, it seems to chase the protesters rather than leading them.

5 The Politicization of COVID-19 Issue by Populists

Since the beginning of the crisis, the German government has been striving to achieve the broadest possible acceptance for its COVID-19 policy. This goal was served by the involvement of the RKI as scientific authority as well as close and consensus-oriented coordination with the governments of the federal states. Both elements can be understood as a strategy of depoliticization. This strategy must be seen in large parts as failed. Because up to the present day, the scope and orientation of the COVID-19 policy are still being debated. The main line of conflict, widely covered by the media, runs between the following positions: One side advocates nationwide uniform standards and typically also advocates more rigid protective measures ('safety first'). The other side advocates a targeted response to acute infections and emphasizes the need for proportionality in dealing with measures that restrict freedom ('individual rights first'). This conflict runs right through the parties, especially in the CDU ('intra-partisan conflict'); it also divides the governments between the Bund and some of the Länder ('intergovernmental conflict') and reflects to some extent the East-West-difference, because it is primarily East German politicians who, due to the small number of COVID-19 cases in their states, are against rigid pandemic policies.

The intergovernmental conflict in particular has consequences for the AfD: First, the intergovernmental line of conflict has led to a kind of permanent politicization of the pandemic, which became even more entrenched after Easter with the increasing replacement of the federal government's leadership role by the Länder. This form of intergovernmental politicization of the pandemic has left little room for the opposition to present itself, and the AfD in particular has hardly had a chance to distinguish itself in the concert of media attention. In addition, the AfD's centre of power is located in the eastern part of the republic, but the two prime ministers of Saxony and Saxony-Anhalt have already been able to successfully present themselves in the media as critics of the federal government.

Initially, the AfD's politicization strategy was strongly aimed at accusing the federal government of incompetence in prevention and crisis management. With this focus of criticism, however, a preliminary decision had already been made on the status of COVID-19: The pandemic is real, as is the virus. Whereas many populists seem to question the biological existence of Corona, the AfD has not been challenging the main elements of the government's COVID-19 narrative. The *naming* and *blaming* is therefore only directed towards the *management by* the government. This led to a path dependency of the argumentation, which basically opened up little scope for castigating the *emergence of* the virus or the pandemic itself as a political problem; for example, as exaggeration on the part of the government or through conspiracy theories. For the AfD as an opposition, a *confrontation* with the state's COVID-19 policy was only possible within the government's narrative of what was necessary, which meant that the criticism lacked clout. For clout is gained through the 'pros and cons' of positions (salience) and not through a 'more or less' within a position (valence).

This open field of criticism of government policy has been occupied by actors of the civil society that apparently pursues the goal of aggregating the growing dissatisfaction and transforming it into a protest movement, possibly a political party. One of these attempts, called 'Resistance 2020', became a non-starter. However, this example illustrates the growing willingness of the COVID-19 'losers' (the retail trade, the solo self-employed and artists, etc.) to demonstrate together with the 'system opposition', i.e. the radical left and extreme right. Not only does a radical refusal to comply with COVID-19 regulations take place in these circles, e.g. in the form of 'Corona parties'. This consensus of non-compliance is also the breeding ground for 'alternative' narratives on the origins of the virus and its spread. Due to the path dependency of its own argumentation, the AfD has so far not been able to establish a sustainable connection to these forms of protest within the civil society.

Such a lasting connection would require a form of *naming* and *blaming* that AfD has not been willing to do so far. With regard to prevention, it demands greater independence for Germany in production of drugs and protective equipment and greater consideration for of 'national interests', and with regard to the COVID-19 restrictions, it advocates a more family-friendly and economy-supportive approach. If the AfD, for example, refers to British studies on the risk of childhood infection in support of a more family-friendly approach, it does not question the scientific basis of COVID-19 in principle, but is instead affirming science-orientation as a basis for the debate. It is no wonder that this kind of *claiming* makes little impression on all those who think COVID-19 is a product of governmental fear politics or simply *fake*. Against this background, it does not come as a surprise that the AfD has changed its position—a strategy that aims at regaining the status as the 'true alternative' to government. It no longer belongs to the camp of the 'safety first' supporters, but to the 'individual rights first' representatives. It is no longer focused on the right measures to protect the population during the crisis, but on the 'Corona measures crisis' (Höchst, 29/05/2020), or simply on the 'lockdown crisis' (e.g. Protschka, 13/05/2020).

In the eyes of AfD politicians, this was a reflex to the state's Corona policy (Spangenberg, 23/04/2020). However, there can be no doubt that the change of position within the AfD itself took place relatively quickly. For example, the co-chair of the parliamentary group Weidel characterized the situation on March 4 in the German Bundestag with the sentence: '*We are at the beginning of a Corona epidemic*' (Weidel, 04/03/2020). A good week later, MP Holm swore that the Germans have to come together in the crisis (Holm, 13/03/2020). And his colleague Hess added concrete demands, including the immediate nationwide closure of all schools and public institutions, a ban on entry of people from high-risk areas and the cancellation of mass events. '*Anyone who does not act decisively now*', said Hess (13/30/2020), 'increases the probability that the crisis will get out of control, as it did in Italy'.

After the Bund and Länder agreed on March 22 on strict COVID-19 measures, the AfD immediately began to change its position towards '*individual rights first*'. '*What alternatives are there to the current course?*' Gauland (25/03/2020), co-chair of the parliamentary group of the AfD, linked his question with the demand for a time limit on protective measures, and argued that the government's policies are excessive and economically damaging. This set the tone for others: In the long run, Jongen said, these measures can neither be financed nor sustained, especially since they ignore the social costs of such crisis management (e.g., 22/04/2020). Therefore, back to normality—the faster, the better (e.g. v. Storch, 07/05/2020). From May onwards, this position was enriched with accusations that the government exploits the COVID-19 measures to pursue other purposes: the desire to distract from past failures (e.g. Hemmelgarn, 13/05/2020); the effort to expand governmental power (Wolfgang Wiehle, 15/05/2020); the plan to push through socialist utopias (Huber, 19/06/2020) or a sell-out of the country (Kotré, 27/05/2020)

Especially the accusations against the government of panic-mongering (e.g. Kotré, 06/05/2020), in order to incapacitate citizens (e.g. Witt,

02/07/2020), were suitable to join the new-APO against the government's COVID-19 policies. So far, the response to this politicization strategy has had no discernible effect. The AfD is not among the winners of the COVID-19 crisis in public opinion (https://www.wahlrecht.de/umfragen/index.htm): To the extent that state institutions, especially the government, have gained in confidence (Forsa, 02/09/2020), the survey results for the AfD are relatively meagre during the pandemic so far.

6 Conclusion

During the past crises, especially during the high time of migration in 2015, the AfD was perceived as the 'true opposition' by many of those who were dissatisfied with the migration and integration policies of the German government. The party succeeded in attracting and mobilizing voters (Geiges 2018), compared to the CSU, because its criticism was always harsher and more extreme in rhetoric and demands than that of other critics. In this polarized field of migration policy this kind of radical approach helped in 'outbidding' the CSU and others because large parts of the citizenry viewed the AfD's performance as authentic and gave the party credit for it, particularly in the eastern parts of Germany. The COVID-19 crisis is different for two reasons.

First, the AfD itself became a victim of 'outbidding' by the APO, since the 'real opposition' takes place outside of parliament in the streets at 'Corona parties' and demonstrations in which many participants are not only criticizing, but resisting the government's Corona policies. Compared to this amount of resistance, the AfD appears to be part of the establishment due to its 'safety first' logic of *naming*, *blaming* and *claiming* in the beginning of the pandemic in Germany, which largely stayed within the government's narrative of the COVID-19 pandemic.

Second, the AfD failed to get the media's attention. In the early phase of the emergence of the pandemic in Germany, this attention was absorbed by the intergovernmental conflict between the different government's Corona positions and policies. Now the media focus has shifted to the non-compliance of the Corona-APO with whom the AfD tries to connect, but without much success in terms of the limelight. However, this can change again relatively quickly, namely if the AfD succeeds in establishing a linkage between the government's Corona policy and the issue of migration (as for the attempts on part of the AfD). The other parties have so far been unable to find a recipe against the AfD's winning theme of migration. The COVID-19 pandemic may have only postponed this problem, but not eliminated it.

References

Geiges, L. (2018). Wie die AfD im Kontext der 'Flüchtlingskrise' mobilisierte. Eine empirische-qualitative Untersuchung der 'Herbstoffensive 2015'. *Zeitschrift für Politikwissenschaft, 28*(1), 49–69.

Ignazi, P. (1992). The Silent Counter-Revolution: Hypotheses on the Emergence of Extreme Right-Wing Parties in Europe. *European Journal of Political Research, 22*(1), 3–34.

Laakso, M., & Taagepera, R. (1979). 'Effective' Number of Parties: A Measure with Application to West Europe. *Comparative Political Studies, 12*(1), 3–27.

Manow, P. (2018). *Die Politische Ökonomie des Populismus*. Berlin: Suhrkamp.

Rosenfelder, J. (2017). Die Programmatik Der AfD: Inwiefern Hat sie sich von einer primär euroskeptischen zu einer rechtspopulistischen Partei entwickelt? *Zeitschrift Für Parlamentsfragen, 48*(1), 123–140.

Sartori, G. (1976). *Parties and Party Systems: A Framework for Analysis*. Cambridge: Cambridge University Press.

CHAPTER 7

Hungary: Crisis as Usual—Populist Governance and the Pandemic

Márton Bene and Zsolt Boda

1 Introduction

Hungary is a special case in the European Union: since 2010 the country is governed by the populist right-wing party coalition of Fidesz and the Kereszténydemokrata Néppárt (Fidesz and Christian Democratic People's Party, KDNP—hereafter referred to as Fidesz since the KDNP plays only a subordinated role). The governance of Fidesz has been long characterized by markedly populist elements like majoritarianism, anti-pluralism and illiberal tendencies, polarizing politics, strong leadership, and a direct communication with the electorate (Bartha et al. 2020). Fidesz has been very active in communication and constant campaigning, conveying a 'populist myth' (Körösényi et al. 2020): the construction of the 'hard-working Hungarian people' coupled with criticism towards the EU, anti-immigration discourse, and adversarial narratives concerning unpopular minorities (LMBTQ people, Gipsies). The pandemic has not

M. Bene · Z. Boda (✉)
Centre for Social Sciences, Budapest, Hungary
e-mail: boda.zsolt@tk.mta.hu

G. Bobba and N. Hubé (eds.), *Populism and the Politicization of the COVID-19 Crisis in Europe*,
https://doi.org/10.1007/978-3-030-66011-6_7

brought about substantially new development in this respect: Fidesz simply adapted its communication patterns and political logic to the circumstances. Migrants have been blamed for the pandemic and the EU for inadequate policies; polarizing narratives have kept being echoed about the political opposition; and the government has made controversial decisions in order to weaken the opposition parties and municipalities governed by them. Prime Minister, Viktor Orbán, has shown strong leadership and health policy measures have been symbolically militarized. However, at the same time the government has not been hostile to medical expertise and the imposed precautionary measures have effectively contained the spread of the disease.

2 Political Context

Since 2010 Hungary has been governed by Fidesz, a right-wing party and its unquestioned leader, Orbán who has been serving as Prime Minister. Since 2010 Fidesz has won three parliamentary elections with a constitutional majority (two-third of the seats) due to four main reasons. First, in 2010 the Hungarian Socialist Party (Magyar Szocialista Párt—MSZP), the leading force of the left, collapsed under corruption charges and the heavy consequences of the 2007–2009 economic crisis. MSZP split under the crisis and in 2010 two new parties, the radical right-wing Jobbik (Jobbik Magyarországért—For a Better Hungary) and the green LMP (Lehet Más a Politika—Another Politics is Possible) also formed groups in the parliament. Since then the fragmented and poorly organized opposition could not propose a convincing political alternative to the rule of Fidesz. Second, the past decade brought about a fast-economic recovery coupled with an increasing inflow of EU-money to Hungary. This has created a favourable economic situation in the country and growing prosperity to large segments of the society. Third, Fidesz has used its comfortable parliamentary majority not only to initiate a series of radical policy changes, but also to alter the system of institutional checks and balances and create illiberal reforms that strengthen its power position. Fidesz unilaterally passed a new constitution and changed the electoral system to its own advantage. Fourth, although the government has not been engaged in 'macroeconomic populism' (Dornbusch and Edwards 1990) and has pursued a rather responsible, or even neoliberal fiscal policy (cutting spending on social benefits, health care, and education) it has managed through a series of well-targeted policy measures and active communication to create legitimacy for its decisions. For instance, the slogan of 'workfare society' legitimized the cutting of unemployment benefits and the introduction of the compulsory public works programme for the unemployed as well as the tying of family support schemes to legal (taxable) income. This policy package has an implicit anti-Gipsy message (Bartha et al. 2020).

Originally a moderate conservative party, in the past decade Fidesz has been gradually radicalizing both in terms of policy positions and communication patterns. Today it has an uncompromising anti-immigration stance, upholds the traditional family model, questions the rights of LMBTQ people, and conveys anti-EU messages sometimes rooted in blatant conspiracy theories. Although Fidesz is member of the European People's Party group in the European Parliament, its membership was suspended as during the 2019 European Parliamentary election campaign the party used posters on which Jean-Claude Juncker, then the president of the European Commission, was portrayed with Hungarian-American billionaire and philanthropist George Soros with the caption: '*You have the right to know what Brussels is up to!*'. Fidesz spends huge amounts on communication and uses various channels. The public broadcasting has become a propaganda channel for the government where politicians of the opposition have practically no chance to be invited to. Through businesspersons close to the government Fidesz controls most of the commercial radio stations, many daily and weekly newspapers and the overwhelming majority of public billboards (Polyák 2019). That is, Hungarian media is characterized by an extreme form of parallelism, with little overlap between the thematization of the pro-governmental and the independent media universes. Besides its active media policy, the government regularly organizes so-called National Consultations in which the citizens are asked about current political issues. However, the results of the National Consultations are not transparent and accountable and the whole institutions are more about conveying manipulative messages than to gather inputs from the people (Batory and Svensson 2019).

While in 2010 Jobbik, a radical right-wing party was its main rival, Fidesz has managed to take over the messages of Jobbik on law and order measures, compulsory public works for the unemployed, cultural war against the liberal elite, extreme nationalism, and hostility towards immigration. Today Jobbik, seriously weakened, seems to be more moderate, more liberal and pro-European than Fidesz.

Fidesz, while dominating the legislation, has been also the strongest party at the local level. At the municipal elections of both 2010 and 2014, it was by far the most successful party gaining majority in all regional councils, winning all (but one: Szeged) of the major cities, including Budapest, the capital city. However, the 2019 municipal elections brought about a breakthrough of the coalition of opposition parties. Although Fidesz remained the most popular party, it was defeated in half of the major cities. Budapest elected Gergely Karácsony, the candidate of the opposition for mayor and the coalition of opposition parties won in most of the districts in the capital city. The key of the success of the opposition was to overcome its fragmentation and create a coalition for the elections. In Hungary, it meant the cooperation of the left-wing, liberal, green and right-wing opposition parties of the opposition. At the local level some other actors, like civil organizations and other, smaller parties have also joined in. It is obvious that these coalitions are extremely fragile and their political survival is far from being evident. Nevertheless, the municipal elections of November 2019 put a dent into the myth of invincibility of Orbán and Fidesz. It is a major political change since 2010 and provides an important element of the political context at the time of pandemic.

It is also important that the critiques of healthcare policy are one of the main topics of the opposition since 2010. They often emphasize that the government neglect healthcare system which is thereby in terrible state. Over the last ten years, several anti-government demonstration and campaign have been organized to protest against the government's healthcare policy. Polls also often show that people perceive the state of healthcare system as the most important problem the country faces (Table 1).[1]

3 COVID-19 Diffusion and Political Measures

As in many other European countries, the government reacted early to the news about the pandemic and set up on January 31 the so-called Operational Group. This government body has been responsible for monitoring the epidemiological situation, coordinating the measures taken as a response to the pandemic and providing the public with the necessary information. The Operational Group held lengthy daily press

[1] E.g. Standard Eurobarometer 92, November 2019, Hungarian country report.

Table 1 Main Hungarian political parties (>5% in the last general election)

Political party	*2018 general election*		*2019 European election*	
	Vote shares[a]	*Seats*	*Vote shares*	*Seats*
In power				
Fidesz – KDNP	49.6%	133	52.6%	13
In opposition				
Jobbik	19.2%	26	6.3%	1
MSZP – PM	13%	20	6.6%	1
DK	5.4%	9	16%	4
LMP	7.1%	8		
Momentum	–	–	9.9%	2

[a]The Hungarian system consists of a combination of individual mandates and party lists. The vote share data refer to the latter
Source valasztas.hu (official resource)

conferences televised real time—however, since the middle of March journalists could not ask questions on the spot, they had to send in their questions beforehand by e-mail. The Operational Group did not answer all questions and especially independent journalists and media outlets have been complaining about no response to their queries.

The first cases of COVID-19 were identified in March. As a response, on March 11 2020, the government declared the state of emergency. From this time on the government issued a series of emergency decrees, in which it partially suspended the application of certain acts as well as enacted new regulations. Arrivals from Italy, China, South Korea and Iran were banned, just like indoor events involving more than 100 and outdoor events involving more than 500 participants. On March 13, the prime minister announced the closure of all kinds of educational institutions. Three days later further restrictive measures were announced by Orbán: the borders of Hungary were closed, so that only Hungarian citizens were allowed to enter the country; all public and social events were banned. From March 27, physical movement of citizens was restricted too.

On March 30, the parliament passed the Coronavirus Act (labelled as Authorization Act) which permitted to the government to rule by decrees without any functional or time limitation, without any debate in the legislation, and without any guarantee for immediate constitutional review. The Act stirred heavy criticisms from both internal and international actors as a potentially damaging move for democracy. MPs of the European Parliament raised concerns about the Act and warned about the rule of law. However, 2.5 months later, on June 16 the parliament called back the Coronavirus Act and the government triumphed over its critics, arguing that people who had accused the government of dictatorship were calumniators. But the same day the parliament also voted for a previously unknown legal order, the so-called health crisis situation in which upon the declaration of the Surgeon General the government acquires special powers again.

From the beginning of April to mid-May Hungary was experiencing the speeding up of local transmission. One of the most significant measures in this period was the ordering of public hospitals to free up 60% of their capacity, equalling 36 thousand beds. On April 7, there were around 800 known cases so the capacity made available largely exceeded the foreseeable need, while rumours were spreading about the dramatic fate of the patients that had been forced to go home. Then and since the political opposition has made several attempts to criticize the hasty decision, but failed to provide convincing evidences about the consequences to the public. From the end of April, the government started to selectively lift lockdown measures, and finally ending the emergency situation on June 16. Overall Hungary has managed to contain the spread of the disease fairly effectively, and the number of both known COVID cases and COVID-related deaths has remained relatively low (see Fig. 1 and Table 2).

As part of the emergency measures, the government introduced a series of decisions aimed at alleviating the economic hardship. These included tax exemptions for small businesses and individual entrepreneurs, the acceleration of VAT refunds to improve the solvency of small- and medium-size enterprises, and the extension of taxation related deadlines. On the other hand, in order to generate additional revenues new surtaxes on credit institutions and the retail sector were introduced, transfers to municipalities and the state subsidies of political parties were curtailed.

While the government started a communication campaign already during the lockdown advertising the governmental measures and their supposed effectiveness the opposition has argued that Hungary, unlike most of the European countries, fell short of providing large-scale subsidies to businesses for the preservation of workplaces and that several targeted financial aids went directly to businesspeople close to the government.

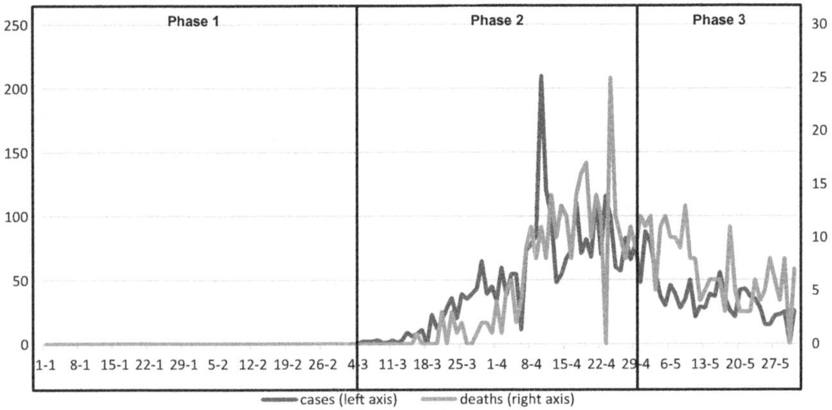

Fig. 1 Daily death toll and new cases in Hungary (*Source* European Centre for Disease Prevention and Control. Phase 1: pre-COVID-19; Phase 2: spread and containment measures; Phase 3: contagion mitigation)

Table 2 COVID-19 pandemic in Hungary

Cases	4027
Total deaths	551
Total recovered	2355
Cases for 1 M pop	417
Deaths for 1 M pop	57

Source www.worldometers.info/coronavirus/ (update 10/6/2020)

4 Populist Discourse at the Time of COVID-19

During the pandemic, the same populist arguments and frames appeared in the communication of the governmental politicians than in normal periods; therefore, the dominant discourse has changed little. As Körösényi et al. (2020) argued there is an overarching narrative behind the communication of the Orbán-regime, the so-called populist myth (Casullo 2020), whose main elements are applied to interpret any major political issue and crisis. The central narrative of this populist myth is that the leader and its people together fight for 'the Hungarians' national interests and freedom against the interconnected international and national enemies who seriously threat these interests and freedom for their own political and economic benefits. This 'populist myth' makes charismatic leadership possible as it creates a charismatic bond between the leader and its followers and maintain the leader's capacity to act in a highly flexible way (Körösényi et al. 2020: 59–61). Orbán's charismatic leadership was a central feature of the Hungarian crisis management (see, Merkovity et al. 2020), and the commonly used elements of this 'populist myth' pervaded the government communication of the crisis. In the construction and dissemination of this discourse, the government communication could also draw upon the centrally organized extensive pro-government media network that uncritically produced and echoed the elements of this narrative.

The 'people' were a constant reference point to the government's, and especially Orbán's communication. During the crisis, people were usually referred as 'Hungarians' as an inclusive but homogenizing label which is a commonly used concept to describe the objects of the political representation in the Orbán-regime. The main official slogans of the crisis communication were '*No Hungarian is alone*' and '*every Hungarian is responsible for every Hungarian*', and Viktor Orbán often discussed and analysed the attributes, behaviour, efforts and performance of the 'Hungarians'. In these talks, Orbán always painted a very favourable picture about 'Hungarians' and describe them as highly disciplined, intelligent, brave, helpful and sympathetic. He also frequently talked about the everyday difficulties 'Hungarians' face during the pandemic in a sympathizing and mundane way showing he knows very well these ordinary problems. For instance, in an interview he told: '(…) *I know exactly that staying home with two or three children (…) is the jihad in itself*'.[2] Beyond these references another way to involve 'the people' into the crisis management was that pro-government think tanks published a lot of polls during the crisis, and their results have become a constant reference point in the pro-government media public to show that 'the people' highly support the governments' measures. To present this support more clearly, in July the government launched a National Consultation where citizens can express their opinion about the crisis management through directed and carefully selected questions. As discussed before, the main function of these National Consultation is to justify popular support for the government's measures and show that the government acts in line with the people's will. The questionnaire included questions about what measures

[2] Radio Kossuth, 04/17/2020.

the government should do in the future (e.g. free Internet for teachers, strengthen the protection of elderly home), but there were items about George Soros ('*Do you reject George Soros's plan, which would put our homeland in debt for an unforeseeably long period of time?*'), immigration, '*hostile foreign acquisition*' of companies by '*international financial speculators*' and Brussels' '*offensive against the immigration-related regulations of the Hungarian constitution*' as closely related issues to the pandemic.[3]

In line with the central narrative of the 'populist myth', the relationship between the incumbent elite and 'the people' is not presented as conflicting, instead their organic unity and cooperation are emphasized. Orbán often stressed that an effective crisis management requires proper collaboration between the incumbent elite and 'the people'. At the same time, strong elite criticism is an important part of the crisis communication, but as a usual element of the prevailing discourse, this is directed to the global, especially the European elites. The major sphere of this anti-elitist rhetoric is the strong international and national critiques of the Coronavirus Act enacted at the end of March. As a response of concerns expressed by international and national actors, the government and its allied media argued that the liberal mainstream including the European political elites, international media outlets, NGOs and their affiliated national allies such as the opposition and the left-liberal media attacked the country and its government who put its all efforts to defend the nation from the pandemic. This attack is politically motivated as this liberal mainstream aims at overthrowing the government and therefore wants to make the crisis management to be unsuccessful. They also highlight that these international and national actors are all connected by being supported by George Soros, the Hungarian-American billionaire, the main enemy of the government. Soros was also accused of using the crisis for his own economic interests with his idea about the perpetual bonds European Union should use to finance the recovery. Orbán referred to this idea as Soros-plan 2.0 which aims at making European Union to be 'debt slavery'. A further recurring claim was in the pro-government media public that the sharp fall in the value of the Hungarian forint in the first weeks of the pandemic was due to Soros's speculative intervention motivated by his own political and

[3] see, About Hungary: Here is the latest national consultation questionnaire in English http://abouthungary.hu/news-in-brief/heres-the-latest-national-consultation-questionnaire-in-english/.

economic interests. European political elites were also highly criticized by pro-government actors for their inefficiency in crisis management. They often argued that Western European countries and the European Union failed in protecting their citizens which was usually contrasted with the Hungarian and Central-Eastern European crisis management presented as highly successful. Overall, these arguments are recurring elements of the dominant pro-government discourse in Hungary, the construction of the politically motivated, interconnected and inefficient European elites is a major ingredient of the 'populist myth' discussed by Körösényi and his colleagues (2020).

At least since 2015 the outgroup in the image of 'immigrants' is also an inherent part of this narrative. However, during the pandemic this element was dominant only in the first weeks of the crisis, later its presence was rather marginal. At this first phase, pro-government actors, including Orbán, often argued that there is a clear link between the pandemic and immigration, and for these reasons the defence of the borders and the rigid immigration policy are crucial to protect 'the Hungarians'. This narrative was amplified by the fact that the first infected cases were students from Iran who were reported to aggressively confront to the protective measures in the hospital and violate quarantine rules. This incident received heightened attention in the pro-government media sphere, and the Operational Group being responsible for the daily information service also intensively reported about it. A few days later the government expelled these students from the country. Later less words were devoted to immigrants by pro-government actors, and though the argument about the link between the pandemic and immigration did not disappear entirely, the topic became marginal in the crisis communication. The Chinese origin of the crisis was not problematized in the government's discourse. Instead, China appeared as a supportive ally who is the main provider of protective equipment owing to the great commercial relationships built up previously by the government.

5 The Politicization of COVID-19 Issue by Populists

Given the fact that populists in Hungary are in governmental position, and the Coronavirus Act gave them even stronger authority, they could easily and immediately enact any idea. In fact, pro-government actors often highlighted that they were able to make and implement the most important decisions much sooner than other countries that is the main reason of the effective crisis management. They also stressed that this effective decision-making was made possible by the highly criticized Coronavirus Act which allowed the PM to manage the crisis personally. In the managing phase, Orbán stated that the Coronavirus Act was his best decision over the last ten years. As the Act is shown as the main force of the successful crisis management, its previous opponents could be easily presented retrospectively as who seriously endangered the effective protection of the people during the pandemic.

However, during the emergence phase the topic of COVID-19 received less attention by pro-government actors. Although preventing measures such as setting up the Operational Group and the acceptance of an Action Plan were made at the end of January, the prime minister kept distance from the topic until the middle of March. As a sign of the depoliticized approach, the issue was managed by lower-level policy makers indicating that the government considered it to be a policy rather than political question. For instance, at the end of February, Orbán missed his usual speech in the opening day of the spring session of the parliament to give the floor to the Minister of Human Resources to talk about the COVID-19 situation, while he told in an interview that '*although the coronavirus is attracting now all the attention, the historical challenge we face is still the migration itself*'.[4] In this period, it was only the opposition that tried to politicize the topic by emphasizing that the healthcare system is not well-prepared for the pandemic which attempts were highly criticized by pro-government politicians and media actors who often accused the opposition politicians and media outlets of overstating the challenge and making panic.

Since the virus appeared in Hungary, this approach has suddenly changed, and the PM has become the clear leader of the crisis management both in the government's communication and the pro-governmental media (see, Merkovity et al. 2020). While this change indicates that the government no longer considered the topic as a pure policy question that should be managed by politicians being responsible for the specific area, their main argument was that the crisis management cannot have a politics aspect. Governmental political actors argued that the crisis management is exclusively about protecting people from the

[4] Rádió Kossuth, 02/28/2020.

medical and economic consequences of the pandemic, and any politics-related interpretation or claim is invalid and harmful from this respect. According to them, the effective crisis management requires national unity and to set aside any political rivalry. This approach is also stressed by comparing the situation to wartime and describing it war-like metaphors.

However, as a reversed form of politicization, this problem-solving approach was attributed only to the government, and any critique of their measures made by the opposition, professional associations such as the Hungarian Medical Chamber or teachers' union, NGOs, experts or media outlets was labelled as politically motivated attack, and pro-government politicians usually highlight their alleged underlying political motives. While this strategy appeared in several issues related to the crisis management, it was the most prominent in case of the national and international controversy about the Coronavirus Act. The pro-government politicians and media actors argued that this law is the most important tool for the effective defence and its exclusive purpose is to make this possible. Its opponents including the international and national political actors, media and NGOs attack it only because they want to make the crisis management unsuccessful as this could result in the fall of the government. To sum up, the 'naming' appeared in a reversed way as the main argument was that while the government manages the crisis as it is without any political motivation, its opponents make strong efforts to politicize the issue in line with their power interests.

The pro-government actors often stressed that their crisis management strongly relied on the opinions of scientists and experts. Orbán also claimed that he is not too familiar with the topic; therefore, he needs to consult with scientists frequently to make reasonable decisions, and on his Facebook page he often showed segments from his meetings with experts. However, he also made it clear that expert opinions are unable to substitute political decisions and drew a definite line between the expert and political knowledge. He argued that expert opinions cannot guide political measures directly as political decisions are more based on the 'common sense' that he owns. Expert opinions serve only as a crucial factual background for these 'common sense'-based political decisions. However, it is also important to note that while Orbán and other pro-government actors often referred to the importance of embracing scientists' knowledge and opinions, these experts were hardly visible in front of the public. The official faces of the information service beyond the Surgeon General of Hungary were from policing bodies therefore people in uniforms were a determining visual feature of the official crisis communication.

In the phase of confrontation, blaming played an important role in the communication of the government. While the government kept highlighting the efficiency of their measures, for the existing problems the newly elected oppositional mayor of the capital city, Karácsony, was mostly blamed. The main object of these critiques was the fact that an elderly care home run by the municipality of Budapest has become the primarily node of the Hungarian pandemic. Pro-government actors and media outlets made Karácsony personally responsible for this incident and argued that his passive and ineffective political leadership and crisis management led to this tragic event. Orbán also strongly blamed the mayor, criticizing sharply his personal leadership quality and abilities, and mentioned that after the crisis his responsibility would be examined in legal way. Naturally, Karácsony kept refusing his personal responsibility for this incident; instead, he argued that some government measures and the lack of proper information-services lead to these infections. Further, it is important to note that Karácsony was already under attack before this incident as his several measures were highly criticized by pro-government actors. Another repeatedly blamed actor was the European Union that was presented as passive, ineffective and unhelpful in the crisis management while highly active in political-motivated attacks against the government. As an evidence for the inefficacy of the European Union, the European Centre for Disease Prevention and Control (ECDC) were often highlighted since it predicted the risk of the pandemic to be moderate in its reports until the middle of February which allegedly set back the effective country-level protections.

6 Conclusion

Hungary is a case of populist governance since 2010. Fidesz and its leader, Viktor Orbán, have been using populist political strategy and populist communication patterns for the past decade or more. This blend of strong leadership, illiberal measures, direct communication with the electorate as well as the construction of the 'populist myth' of the strong community of Hungarians versus hostile liberal elites and their protégés, the immigrants were simply adapted to the circumstances of the pandemic. While the government hold that the effective containment of the disease is a national challenge that should not be politicized, any criticism coming from social or political actors were immediately labelled as 'political'. However, a small, but important detail is that Orbán, unlike other populist leaders like Bolsonaro or Trump, never questioned the importance of expert knowledge. At the same time his relationship to expertise has been somewhat ambiguous: medical experts have not been pushed in the forefront of communication with the public and Orbán made clear several times that decisions have to be made by politicians who ultimately rely on their instinct and the common sense.

References

Bartha, A., Boda, Z., & Szikra, D. (2020). When Populist Leaders Govern: Conceptualizing Populism in Policy Making. *Politics and Governance*, *8*(3), 71–81.

Batory, A., & Svensson, S. (2019). The Use and Abuse of Participatory Governance by Populist Governments. *Policy & Politics, 47*(2), 227–244.

Casullo, M. E. (2020). Populism and Myth (25–38). In E. Eklundh, & A. Knott (Eds.), *The Populist Manifesto*. London: Rowman & Littlefield.

Dornbusch, R., & Edwards, S. (1990). Macroeconomic Populism. *Journal of Development Economics, 32*(2), 247–277.

Körösényi, A., Illés, G., & Gyulai, A. (2020). *The Orbán Regime: Plebiscitary Leader Democracy in the Making*. London: Routledge.

Merkovity, N., Bene, M., & Farkas, X. (2020). Hungary. In D. Lilleker, I. Coman, M. Gregor, & E. Novelli (Eds.), *Political Communication and Covid-19: Governance and Rhetoric in Times of Crisis*. London: Routledge (in press).

Polyák, G. (2019). Media in Hungary: Three Pillars of an Illiberal Democracy (279–303). In E. Połońska & C. Beckett (Eds.), *Public Service Broadcasting and Media Systems in Troubled European Democracies*. Cham: Palgrave Macmillan.

CHAPTER 8

Czech Republic: Running the State Like a Family Business

Ondřej Císař and Michal Kubát

1 Introduction

Populism has become a 'new and ubiquitous dimension of politics' (Zanatta 2013) and we may very well be living in the 'epoch of populism' (Liogier 2013). This is not just a general argument; it also applies to the contemporary Czech Republic, where, after being on the margins, it became part of the political mainstream after 2015 (Císař and Štětka 2017). Our chapter considers three parties that display populist features: the ruling party ANO 2011 (ANO) and two non-governmental parties, Freedom and Direct Democracy (Svoboda a přímá demokracie—SPD) and the Communist Party of Bohemia and Moravia (Komunistická strana Čech a Moravy—KSČM), which nevertheless both often back the government in the parliament, KSČM officially. Embodying different faces of populism, all three represent different versions of what the mainstream literature labels as populist parties. This chapter shows that the current

O. Císař · M. Kubát (✉)
Charles University, Prague, Czechia
e-mail: michal.kubat@fsv.cuni.cz

G. Bobba and N. Hubé (eds.), *Populism and the Politicization of the COVID-19 Crisis in Europe*,
https://doi.org/10.1007/978-3-030-66011-6_8

crisis has not yet transformed their rhetoric but has brought to light its most important features. In our text, we first explain the broader political context, the spread of COVID-19 and the political measures to address the virus in the Czech Republic. It looks at the populist discourse of the three parties and, finally, their strategies of (de)politicization regarding the COVID-19 issue. In the case of ANO especially, there was a strong tendency to try to depoliticise the issue by involving experts and especially epidemiologists in the discussion.

2 Political Context

The most successful Czech populist party has been the ANO party. It was established in 2011–2012 and enjoyed a fair amount of success from early on. In the 2013 parliamentary elections, ANO gained 18.65% of the votes and 23.5% of the seats.[1] The movement became part of the government of the Social Democrats, while its founder, sponsor, and unquestioned leader, Andrej Babiš, a billionaire entrepreneur, became Minister of Finance. ANO won the subsequent 2017 parliamentary elections, receiving 29.64% of the votes and 39% of the seats, and became the strongest party. It is then that Babiš, winner of the elections, became Prime Minister.

The second populist party—the SPD—was formed in 2015. It was founded by a Czech-Japanese businessman, Tomio Okamura, who had previously disbanded his first party, Dawn of Direct Democracy (Úsvit přímé demokracie—ÚPD). To some extent, Okamura established his second movement 'just in time', in that the immigrant crisis had just started to flare, and that mobilised not only the SPD but the whole populist political scene (Císař and Navrátil 2019). In the parliamentary elections of 2017, SPD entered the Chamber of Deputies with 10.64% of the votes and 11% of the seats.

What binds and what differentiates these two populist parties? ANO is an 'extreme form of a business-firm party' (Kopeček 2016), which is heavily dependent on its leader (Kubát and Hartliński 2019). It was established at the initiative of its leader as a kind of 'personal vehicle' (Lucardie 2000) that serves the leader as a means of fulfilling his ambitions and needs. While SPD is also a business-firm party, it is not as much

[1] The source of this and following electoral data is the Czech Statistical Office: https://volby.cz/.

a business-firm party as ANO is. Both parties present themselves as anti-establishment and anti-elitist and focus on the alleged ubiquitousness of political corruption. While they have many shared features, the two parties are not identical. While ANO represents an anti-political (rejecting 'traditional corrupted parties') and technocratic or expert form of populism ('experts' should rule instead of 'incompetent politicians'), SPD is clearly professing far-right nationalism and xenophobia (Balík et al. 2019; Císař and Navrátil 2019; Kopeček et al. 2018).

KSČM represents a different case, both in terms of how the party was established and how it evolved in time, and in terms of its political identity and orientation. KSČM is the direct successor of the Communist Party of Czechoslovakia (Komunistická strana Československa—KSČ), which was founded in 1921 and from 1948 to 1989 was the ruling hegemonic party in Czechoslovakia. After the fall of communism in 1989, the party changed its name but, in the end, failed to shed its Marxist-Leninist identity. It never transformed itself into a non-communist socialist or social democratic party (Kunštát 2013). Nevertheless, KSČM has been the most stable Czech party since 1989. Its electoral support has long been around 10–15%, falling to 7.76% only in the last parliamentary elections in 2017. KSČM has never directly participated in any governmental coalition since 1989; however, following the 2017 elections, it became part of a pro-government parliamentary alliance.

KSČM can be described as a 'non-exclusively populist party' (Havlík and Pinková 2012: 29), in which populism is accompanied by another clear set of ideological preferences, in this case vulgar Marxism-Leninism. KSČM is a dogmatic Marxist-Leninist party, nostalgic for the *ancient regime*. It is an anti-system party according to Sartori's (1976: 138) narrow definition of the concept. But can it be classified as a populist party? While KSČM does not fulfil all the defining features of populism, from a longitudinal perspective we can detect strong social populism in its programme (Císař and Štětka 2017; Havlík 2012) and that populism is linked to nationalism. It is a combination of social and national protest (Kubát 2016) (Table 1).

3 COVID-19 Diffusion and Political Measures

News about the global spread of COVID-19 reached the Czech Republic before any individuals tested positive for the virus in the country. In the *first 'pre-COVID-19' phase*, for months the Czech media followed the

Table 1 Main Czech political parties (>5% in the last general election)

Political party	*2017 general election*		*2019 European election*	
	Vote shares	*Seats*	*Vote shares*	*Seats*
In power				
ANO	29.64	78	21.18	6
Communist Party of Bohemia and Moravia[a]	7.76	15	6.94	1
Czech Social Democratic Party	7.27	15	3.95	0
In opposition				
Civic Democratic Party	11.32	25	14.54	4
Czech Pirate Party	10.79	22	13.95	3
Freedom and Direct Democracy	10.64	2	9.14	2
Christian and Democratic Union – Czechoslovak People's Party	5.80	1	7.24	2
TOP 09	5.31	7	11.65[b]	3[b]
Mayors and Independents	5.18	6		

[a]Communist party is not a part of the cabinet, but it supports it in the parliament
[b]Electoral coalition of TOP 09 and Mayors and Independents

situation in China and northern Italy, especially as the latter is a popular vacation spot for many Czechs. Despite the mounting information, the Czech government did not take any serious action until the country had its first positive cases on March 1, 2020.

All the key measures that were supposed to slow down the spread of the COVID-19 were taken during March, when the *second phase* of the epidemic started. Initially, at the beginning of March, travel conditions were tightened and quarantine was introduced for Czech citizens returning from high-risk areas. On March 11, all schools were closed. The following day, the government declared a state of emergency, which, among other things, restricted free movement of people. Most shops and all restaurants were closed on March 14, the state borders were closed on March 16, and wearing masks in public was made mandatory on March 19.[2]

[2]A list of all the measures taken by the Czech government is available on a special website set up by the Ministry of Health of the Czech Republic: https://koronavirus.mzcr.cz.

The Czech Republic was ultimately only mildly impacted by the first wave of the epidemic (see Fig. 1 and Table 2), and most hospital emergency beds were never occupied. Therefore, after the country entered the *third phase* of the epidemic (the mitigation of contagion) early on, by April 14, 2020, the government approved a five-stage plan, during which it gradually lifted most of the measures introduced earlier. Life in the country, with some exceptions, returned to a new normal.

During the state of emergency, a number of problems, controversies, and discussions arose, three of which were the most noticeable. However, none of them globally posed a serious challenge to the government's strategy to fight COVID-19. The first controversy emerged right at the

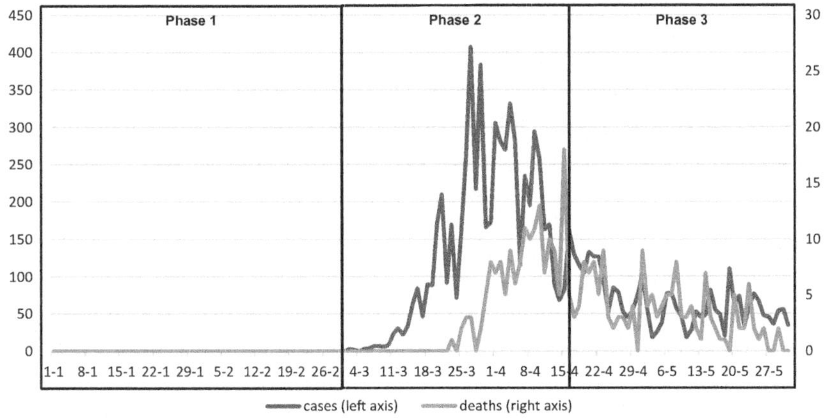

Fig. 1 Daily death toll and new cases in Czech Republic (*Source* European Centre for Disease Prevention and Control. Phase 1: pre-COVID-19; Phase 2: spread and containment measures; Phase 3: contagion mitigation)

Table 2 COVID-19 pandemic in France

Cases	9787
Total deaths	330
Total recovered	7111
Cases for 1 M pop	914
Deaths for 1 M pop	31

Source www.worldometers.info/coronavirus/ (update 10/6/2020)

beginning of the epidemic and was related to the purchase and distribution of medical protective equipment for health professionals. There was a lack of personal protective equipment and their distribution to medical and social facilities was both limited and disorganised. The situation with masks (or their lack of) was characteristic. Sewing masks at home and self-distributing them not only to family members and friends but also to nurses and doctors became a society-wide phenomenon.

The issue of purchasing medical protective equipment also had a strong political line. While some countries, including Taiwan, donated personal protective equipment to the Czech Republic, the government bought most of it in China and at exorbitant prices. The opposition criticised the government on two accounts. First, for favouring expensive and opaquely transacted purchases from China over inciting Czech production. Second, for its responses, as, according to the opposition, the government showed devotion to China but failed to thank Taiwan enough.

The second controversy, which mostly unfolded among different experts, revolved around what constituted appropriate epidemiological measures. The essence of the dispute was that the experts (epidemiologists, biologists, and other medical professionals) themselves disagreed on the most basic points: what caused the COVID-19, how dangerous COVID-19 really is, and whether we were in the midst of a pandemic or not. Related to this were the differing views of experts and also of the public on the country's lockdown, and then also on the gradual lifting of restrictions. The critics of strict measures, mostly various types of experts, pointed out that the country's lockdown would have far worse social and economic and ultimately health (neglecting preventive medical care) effects than the epidemic itself.

Related to this is the economic impact of the crisis, which is the third central point around which debate has revolved. The government recently approved the highest budget deficit in the country's history (up to CZK 500 billion)[3] and the expected economic downturn is [and the economy is expected to shrink by] between 5.5 and 6.5%[4] or even as much as 8%.[5] The crisis has hit tourism and related areas (restaurants and pubs, hotel

[3] Vláda schválila schodek rozpočtu 500 miliard. *Novinky.cz*, 8/06/2020.

[4] Skvělý rok Netflixu i obří ekonomický pokles. Projděte si rekordy kolem koronaviru. *Aktualne.cz*, 2/05/2020.

[5] European Commission. Economic and financial affairs website, Czech Republic.

industry) the most, as well as the automobile industry, which is important for the Czech economy. The opposition disagreed with the measures that the government introduced to boost the economy.

4 Populist Discourse at the Time of COVID-19

In general, Czech political parties that display populist features have not transformed their rhetoric in their reaction to the COVID-19 crisis. There were no substantial changes in the discourse of Prime Minister Babiš and other representatives of his political organisation ANO. In fact, the same symbolism, slogans, and public displays of his direct relationship with the people and its immediate needs have been used during the COVID-19 crisis as were used before it. In fact, Babiš stressed that the crisis provided him with a real opportunity to actually put his signature slogan in practice. In an interview that he gave ten days after the state of emergency was declared, Babiš said: 'We work twenty hours a day, now we are really running the country like a company, just as when there are floods or there is an accident in a chemical factory. So, online, with immediate decisions and implementation. We are now one family, so we run it like a family business with a population of 10.7 million'.[6] After the first wave of the crisis was over, Babiš repeated this stress on company-like effectiveness, his hard-working nature, and his direct and unmediated relationship with the people: 'The coronavirus changed the scope of work of the government and we ultimately managed it like a family company, and it was effective, it was concrete, we saw our decisions in practice. I was at work from morning to night, it was crisis management and it's continuing'.[7]

Instead of changes, there were continuities and specific adaptations in Babiš's communication style and discourse. Before the crisis, Babiš regularly stressed his relationship to the needs of ordinary and/or hard-working people. Unlike his predecessors, he would walk out to meet demonstrators in front of the Governmental Office or would personally visit a hackathon that was organised to protest a particular policy of his government and come up with an alternative IT solution. He stylised himself into the role of both a capable manager and the caring father

[6] Teď řídím stát jako firmu. Ale demokracii neomezím, říká Babiš. *Idnes.cz*, 22/03/2020.

[7] Koronavirus mi umožnil řídit stát jako rodinnou firmu, řekl Babiš. *Idnes.cz*, 7/05/2020.

of the nation, for which image he drew on the historical figure of 'Jan Antonín Baťa, the interwar shoe magnate who had extensive (but never realised) plans in the 1930s to remake the country using management and business techniques' (Hanley and Vachudova 2018: 282). Baťa is also remembered for his direct management methods and the programmes and benefits he introduced to support his employees. During the crisis, this political style was further applied when, for example, Babiš himself visited a food warehouse to check out the availability of basic food items for stores. The same pattern was in place when Babiš, with other members of his cabinet, personally welcomed a cargo plane full of masks and respirators from China at Prague airport.

Babiš's relationship to the European Union, or some of its institutions, is complicated and was so even before the crisis. Although ANO and Babiš support the EU in principle, and mostly as an important source of money for the Czech economy in general, and his holding company in particular, Babiš criticised the EU for its alleged lack of effectivity and capacity for action in the past, especially in relation to the proposals to introduce a permanent EU relocation mechanism as a solution to the 2015 migration crisis. As early as the end of January 2020, he targeted the EU for its lack of activity in relation to the coming coronavirus crisis: '*…unless something fundamental happens, because Europe isn't being very active yet, I'll suggest to the government on Monday that we temporarily ban all flights from China*'.[8] The EU and its policies have been criticised many times since then—for example, when Babiš did not want to support the proposed EU economic recovery plan.

Our observation about the continuity of populist rhetoric also applies to Tomio Okamura's nationalist and far-right SPD. The main target of this party's rhetoric has been the EU, which, according to Okamura, failed in its response to the pandemic. The SPD alleged that the EU was unable to deal with the current crisis in the same way that it failed to cope with the 2015 migration crisis; in the party discourse the two crises are moreover connected to each other. In fact, according to SPD both crises are actively co-created by the EU, which is inviting migrants to the EU as well as forcing individual countries to be dependent on each other in terms of goods and especially food supply. This makes it difficult for individual countries to adequately deal with current challenges, including

[8] Česko kvůli koronaviru rozšíří opatření na letištích. *Česká televize*, 30/01/2020.

the COVID-19 crisis. The party sees food self-sufficiency as the ideal and in fact it wants the country's agricultural and, as much as possible also, its economic system to be autarchic, which it contends is the only way to fight current global problems such as migration and the pandemic. In the view of the party: '*The EU does not help, it does harm. The sooner we leave it, the better*'.[9] The party has actively utilised the COVID-19 crisis to advance its traditional political programme and its focal points such as fight against so-called unadaptable people, or against support for what the party deems 'political' NGOs. It wants any public funding in these areas to be cut and redirected to those who really need the support. The same applies to public support for alternative sources of energy and the planned acquisition of military equipment, which should be stopped or postponed.

KSČM has also continued its pre-crisis nationalist rhetoric. In general, as its Parliamentary supporter, the party was not very critical of the government, with the exception of what the communists saw as the possibly 'endless' extension of the state of emergency. Like the SPD, the party stressed the issue of self-sufficiency, concerning not only food but other strategic commodities as well. The party's traditional fight against globalisation and internationalisation had, in its view, been made even more urgent by the pandemic. Therefore, a strong state, less international economic dependency, and more economic self-sufficiency have become even more important in recent times than before. KSČM also criticised the planned acquisition of military equipment, but mostly on the grounds that it would contribute to an upgrading of NATO, which is an established target for the party. In general, the international environment has represented a traditional source of threat for the party, which was again proven by the current crisis. The most important imperative remains the same as before the pandemic, i.e. not to lose sovereignty and to fight international capital: '*Either developments will be directed in favour of foreign capital, which wants to concentrate more assets and its power in the crisis, or in favour of our citizens. By supporting further growth in wages and social benefits, despite the debt we are not relinquishing control of our economy to foreign capital at this stage*'.[10]

[9] SPD. See: https://spd.cz/eu-chce-pretvorit-evropske-instituce/.

[10] KSČM. See: https://www.kscm.cz/cs/aktualne/aktuality/kscm-jedna-pri-krizi-konstruktivne.

5 The Politicization of the COVID-19 Issue by Populists

As described above, in the first phase, the situation in China and Italy was covered by the Czech media and political actors. In the beginning, the media played an important role in setting the agenda of the COVID-19 issue. Regarding concrete measures, direct flights to China were discontinued as early as the beginning of February, more than a month before the start of the real confrontation phase. However, at the very same time, the Minister of Health (nominated by ANO), Adam Vojtěch, published an article that explicitly downplayed the seriousness of COVID-19, comparing it and its lethality to what he alleged to be the more dangerous 'common' flu and asking the public to calm down: '*Let's hope that the coronaviral and media hysteria will soon disappear, the public will realise that we are not in a [catastrophe] film, and we will return to earth. However, the coronavirus did yield one positive thing. People have begun to pay more attention to flu prevention, actually unwittingly*'.[11] The by now infamous article reiterated what official political representatives were stressing at that time, namely that the country was indeed prepared to deal with the infection should it eventually appear in the country. Only a couple of days before, on January 28, Bohuslav Svoboda, a gynaecologist by profession, and a well-known politician and opposition MP from the Civic Democratic Party (Občanská demokratická strana—ODS), tried unsuccessfully to initiate a discussion in Parliament of COVID-19 and the country's preparedness to cope with it.

The confrontation phase started in mid-March. Since ANO is the governing and strongest party in the country, it was actually in the position to react to and solve the COVID-19 crisis. The measures were adopted in March (see above), based on information from countries already dealing with infections, especially Italy, and only after COVID-19 had arrived to the country. In terms of politicization, we were actually able to observe the opposite trend in ANO's discourse, as it attempted to depoliticise the issue by stressing the role played by experts, especially epidemiologists, in devising policy. Roman Prymula, the non-partisan deputy minister of care and also an epidemiologist, was originally appointed the head of the crisis management team, and politicians made

[11] Ministry of Health of the Czech Republic. See: http://www.mzcr.cz/dokumenty/ceska-koronaviralni-chripka_18483_3693_1.html.

repeated declarations of their reliance on expertise. When announcing the state of emergency, Babiš stressed: '*For me, Mr Prymula and his team are the greatest experts. I'm constantly in touch with him, online. The World Health Organization woke up and said there is a pandemic, and Mr Prymula already told me this a week ago*'.[12]

Babiš repeatedly stressed that the decisions about what anti-COVID-19 measures were introduced were based entirely on the expert knowledge of epidemiologists, so much so that he even said that epidemiologists were the ones actually making the decisions at the peak of the crisis. Although Prymula resisted such claims, he did confirm that during the first two months of the pandemic epidemiologists had a big influence on decision-making and nobody questioned their recommendations.[13] Like some other countries, experts received considerable public support from the population in the midst of the crisis. There was also nearly unanimous political support for the government's general anti-virus measures when they were introduced in March. No visible or substantial criticism from the opposition was formulated in this period; this only occurred later on and was directed at the government's economic recovery plan and, before that, its strategy to acquire protective equipment mostly from China, but was not aimed at the government's general measures to prevent COVID-19 from spreading in the country.

The third phase started in mid-April, when the government approved a five-stage plan to gradually lift the anti-COVID-19 measures that had been introduced and started to discuss and propose measures to help the economy recover. At this stage, the debate focused on a number of issues relating to what types of measures should be introduced and what the adequate extent of these measures should be. These measures were introduced gradually and were often revised on the basis of opposition criticism. It is not our aim here to cover these debates in detail, but we can say that the main dispute was over the state's fiscal strategy. Unlike the previous government and its strategy during the financial crisis, the current government has repeatedly rejected austerity policies and budget cuts, and, on the contrary, it intends to run an exceptionally big budget

[12] Řídí operaci, jakou Česko ještě nezažilo. *Deník N*, 18/03/2020.

[13] Prymula: Epidemie vesele pokračuje, byl bych teď tvrdší, Maďar není odborník. *Reflex*, 8/07/2020.

deficit in order to support public investment and pro-employment policies and to save the economy from a severe recession.

Although there is no principal opposition to this strategy, the government has nevertheless been criticised for its unwillingness to find possible savings in state expenses. Another general critical argument concerns the lack of a more strategic plan on how to tackle the increased deficit and how to consolidate public finances in the future. Critics have pointed to the possible mismanagement of public funds. When the record budget deficit was approved in Parliament on June 8, the condition that KSČM presented to the government in exchange for its support was that the government prepare a plan for fiscal consolidation by the end of September 2020.

A dispute over who was responsible for COVID-19 has been going on mostly outside the arena of party politics and rather on the Internet and social media since the beginning of the pandemic. There are analyses available that monitor the activities of disinformation webs spreading fake news about the fabricated nature of COVID-19 and singling out those who are supposedly responsible for it, whether it be the Chinese or US-based government actors. Out of the parties covered in this chapter, KSČM has probably come closest to entering this discussion in its attempt to clear China of possible responsibility for the pandemic: '*The current historical turning point is caused by the so-called coronavirus pandemic, and all analysts are investigating whether it is an artificial problem or whether it is a problem that is really a part of society's development, who is behind it, and how to evaluate it*'.[14] There is also an EMP from the SPD party who runs one of these disinformation webs, one on which the possibility of COVID-19 being a biological weapon was debated.

6 Conclusion

This chapter has reviewed and discussed the measures adopted by Czech political representatives and their discourse relating to COVID-19: the ruling ANO party and two non-governmental parties, SPD and the KSČM. All three represent different versions of what the mainstream literature labels as populist political parties. The chapter most importantly shows that the current crisis has not yet transformed their rhetoric, but

[14] KSČM. See: https://www.kscm.cz/cs/aktualne/aktuality/politicky-souboj-o-uzemi-cr-se-vyhrocuje.

has had the effect of amplifying the most important components of that rhetoric. For example, in the case of ANO, the managerial approach to governance has been discursively wielded as the single most important tool for fighting COVID-19. The chapter also distinguished three phases of action and discourse relating to the pandemic: emergence, confrontation, and management. In the confrontation phase especially there was a strong tendency to depoliticise the issue by involving experts, especially epidemiologists.

Thus far, the crisis has not had any significant effect on support for political parties in the Czech Republic.[15] The three parties covered here have seen their political support left almost unchanged, and while there was a small but temporary increase in support for ANO and its coalition partner, on the whole there has been no change in the balance of power in the country. Finalising this chapter at the end of July 2020, we can conclude that there is no party that has yet either benefited or lost support due to the crisis.

References

Balík, S. et al. (2019). *Od Palackého k Babišovi. Česká politika 19. až 21. století*. Praha: Dokořán–Masarykova univerzita.

Císař, O., & Navrátil, J. (2019). For the People, By the People? The Czech Radical and Populist Right After the Refugee Crisis (184–198). In M. Caiani & O. Císař (Eds.), *Radical Right Movement Parties in Europe*. London and New York: Routledge.

Císař, O., & Štětka, V. (2017). Czech Republic: The Rise of Populism from the Fringes to the Mainstream (285–298). In T. Aalberg, F. Esser, C. Reinemann, J. Strömbäck, & C. de Vreese (Eds.), *Populist Political Communication in Europe*. London and New York: Routledge.

Hanley, S., & Vachudova, M. (2018). Understanding the Illiberal Turn: Democratic Backsliding in the Czech Republic. *East European Politics, 34*(3), 276–296.

Havlík, V. (2012). The Czech Republic (97–134). In V. Havlík et al. (Eds.), *Populist Political Parties in East-Central Europe*. Brno: MuniPress.

Havlík, V., & Pinková, A. (2012). Seeking a Theoretical Framework: How to Define and Identify Populist Parties? (17–38). In V. Havlík et al. (Eds.), *Populist Political Parties in East-Central Europe*. Brno: MuniPress.

[15] Source: https://www.politico.eu/europe-poll-of-polls/czech-republic/.

Kopeček, L. (2016). I'm Paying, So I Decide: Czech ANO as an Extreme Form of a Business-Firm Party. *East European Politics and Societies, 30*(4), 725–749.

Kopeček, L., et al. (2018). *Já platím, já rozhoduji! Političtí podnikatelé a jejich strany*. Brno: B&P Publishing.

Kubát, M. (2016). Komunistyczna Partia Czech i Moraw – skuteczne połączenie protestu socjalnego i nacjonalistycznego. *Polityka i Społeczeństwo, 14*(1), 79–90.

Kubát, M., & Hartliński, M. (2019). Party Leaders in the Czech Populist Parties and Movements. *Polish Political Science Review, 7*(1), 107–119.

Kunštát, D. (2013). *Za rudou oponou. Komunisté a jejich voliči po roce 1989*. Praha: Sociologické nakladatelství.

Liogier, R. (2013). *Ce populisme qui vient*. Paris: Textuel.

Lucardie, P. (2000). Prophets, Purifiers and Prolocutors: Toward a Theory of the Emergence of New Parties. *Party Politics, 6*(2), 175–185.

Sartori, G. (1976). *Parties and Party Systems: A Framework for Analysis*. Cambridge: Cambridge University Press.

Zanatta, L. (2013). *Il populismo*. Roma: Carocci.

CHAPTER 9

Poland: 'If We Don't Elect the President, the Country Will Plunge into Chaos'

Artur Lipiński

1 Introduction

When the COVID-19 pandemic hit Poland during the presidential campaign (elections had been scheduled for the 10th of May), all political parties were completely focused on the electoral competition and the health crisis was, to a large extent, overshadowed by other issues. The stakes were high. For Law and Justice (Prawo i Sprawiedliwość – PiS), the victory of its candidate, incumbent *Andrzej* Duda, would allow the party to advance its radical reforms (e.g., continue the controversial reforms of the judiciary and impose limits on media freedom); for the oppositional Confederation (Konfederacja), the smallest group in parliament, a good electoral result of its candidate Krzysztof Bosak could provide an opportunity to promote its party radical agenda (i.e., anti-LGBTQ, euro-rejectionist, anti-Semitic, and xenophobic slogans) and would be a good starting point for future parliamentary elections. PiS used the health crisis

A. Lipiński (✉)
Adam Mickiewicz University, Poznań, Poland
e-mail: artur.lipinski@amu.edu.pl

G. Bobba and N. Hubé (eds.), *Populism and the Politicization of the COVID-19 Crisis in Europe*,
https://doi.org/10.1007/978-3-030-66011-6_9

to present its leadership as skillful and competent and their decisions as non-political. They also tried to take advantage of the uneven political field created by the pre-emptive COVID-19 measures which had imposed limits on the campaigns of opposition candidates. However, the health crisis and its economic consequences also had drawbacks for the incumbents and opened a window of opportunity for all opposition parties, including Confederation.

The aim of the paper is to elucidate how PiS and Confederation, two right-wing populist parties who differed in their institutional positions, dealt with the double challenge of the COVID-19 crisis and the presidential elections during a pandemic. It presents the political context, the evolution of pre-emptive measures and policies used to prevent the spread of COVID-19, discursive reactions of the parties, and their strategic decision on how and when to introduce and construct the pandemic as a political issue.

2 Political Context

The genesis of the dominant position of PiS on the Polish political scene may be traced back to its success in the presidential and parliamentary elections of 2005, which allowed it to form a government and decisively increased the salience of its right-wing populist message (Pankowski 2011; Stanley and Cześnik 2019). Since its very beginning in 2001, the core of PiS' agenda was constituted by the idea of a strong state and focus on fighting corruption which underpinned its calls for the 'decommunization' of the state (Lipiński 2016). According to the party's causal story (Stone 1989), the Polish transformation was a result of a collusion between the communist and liberal elites in 1989, which not only affected the quality of the newly-born Polish democracy and free-market economy, but also brought about a climate of moral disease in social life. This agenda helped PiS get into parliament in 2001 and form a government in 2005. As the major opposition party, following its premature loss of power in 2007, PiS continued to employ the populist division between the nation and the establishment and constructed the crisis, particularly following the Smolensk catastrophe in 2010 (Moffitt 2015). Incessantly accusing Donald Tusk's government of ruining the country and weakening its sovereignty in the international arena, they managed a double electoral victory in the 2015 presidential and parliamentary elections, resulting in *235* out of 430 seats in the lower chamber of parliament. The extensive social spending programs implemented by the PiS-led government helped generate considerable political support and helped the party to portray itself as making good on electoral promises and proving more effective than its liberal predecessors.

In the 2019 European Parliament (EP) elections and in the subsequent parliamentary elections later that year, PiS and its minor coalition partners (the United Right) secured a dominant position (45.4% of votes, and 43.59% of votes with 235 seats, accordingly) thanks to a campaign filled with homophobic slogans and criticisms of 'gender ideology', assisted by generous social spending framed as a people-oriented 'revolution of dignity'. This was not, however, an out-and-out victory as PiS lost its majority in the Senate, the upper chamber of parliament with the power to slow down the legislative process. The loss of the Senate increased the importance of the presidential elections planned for May 2020 and the necessity to secure the re-election of Duda. Otherwise, challenged by the Senate and a president with veto power, PiS would not be able to continue its radical policies. At this time, it seemed that the political efforts of the ruling camp and the attention of the public would be entirely focused on this task in the forthcoming months. The emergence of COVID-19 and its potentially adverse outcomes for the incumbents only raised the stakes of the elections and determined PiS's resistance to delay the election date.

Another important result of the October 2019 elections was the relative success of Confederation, a radical right-wing party founded at the beginning of 2019 on the eve of an electoral campaign for the European and national parliaments, with 11 seats won in the latter (6.81% of votes). The party showed its ability to surpass PiS from the right flank and succeeded in forcing PiS to radicalize its message. Confederation's anti-systemic agenda makes it similar to many small and short-lived parties which appeared in Poland after 1989, using presidential elections as an opportunity structure to promote a radical message and relying on their 'newness' as an important symbolic resource (Sikk 2012). In general, Confederation is a coalition of economic libertarians linked to the eccentric Janusz Korwin-Mikke and nationalists from the National Movement. During the 2019 EP elections, the coalition was broadened to include anti-vaccine and pro-life activists. The populist strategy of provocation was articulated through anti-Semitic slogans related to the alleged Jewish wartime reparation claims enabled by the American JUST Act of 2017. Moreover, the campaign resorted to anti-Semitic and Eurosceptic slogans to accuse PiS of undermining Poland's sovereignty by becoming servile

Table 1 Poland's Main political parties (>5% in the last general election)

Political party	*2019 General election*		*2019 European election*	
	Vote shares	*Seats*	*Vote shares*	*Seats*
In power				
PiS	43.59%	235	45.38%	26
In opposition				
Civic Coalition (PO, Modern, PL Greens)[a]	27.4%	134	38.47%	22
Democratic Left Alliance[b]	12.56%	49	–	–
Polish People's Party[b]	8.55%	30	–	–
Confederation 'Freedom and Independence'	6.81%	11	4.55%	0

[a]In the 2019 European Parliamentary elections, it started as a European Coalition together with the Polish People's Party and Democratic Left Alliance
[b]Initially as a part of European Coalition

towards the US and EU. Following a failure to reach the 5% parliamentary representation threshold for parties (they only received 4.6% of the votes), Confederation decided to significantly moderate its public image. In the subsequent parliamentary elections in October 2019, they presented themselves as the only integral right-wing force, in comparison with PiS who were shown as lacking in a real right-wing identity. Consequently, Confederation's focus on anti-establishment messages, tax reductions, and other free-market slogans coupled with careful avoidance of more controversial issues brought them 11 seats in parliament (Table 1).

3 COVID-19 Diffusion and Political Measures

In Poland, the pre-COVID phase which lasted until the 4th of March was already marked by the widespread awareness of the seriousness of the health consequences of contracting the virus and the strong strain this would put on health systems in countries affected by the epidemic. The crisis management team at the Ministry of Health met for the first time on the 29th of January. In February, the government took a number of precautionary measures, including formalizing the team monitoring the COVID-19 epidemiological situation.[1] A special act decreed on the 3rd of March outlined emergency powers and responsibilities for public servants and businesses.[2] Importantly, the law was voted for almost unanimously, with Confederation being the only party which opposed it. In general, the government focused on monitoring, informing, and adopting a number of preventive measures.

The second phase of the state's response to the pandemic was triggered by the first case of infection, announced on the 4th of March by the Ministry of Health. On March 10th, i.e., six days after the first case, the government introduced significant limits on mass events. Between the 10th and 12th of March, further lockdown measures were taken, including the closure of schools and universities. A state of epidemic threat was announced on March 14th, two days after the first death from COVID-19. It allowed the Minister of Health to introduce further measures to limit the movement of people. Declaring a state of epidemic threat allowed for an entry ban on foreigners, 14-day quarantine for Poles returning from abroad, limits on gatherings of over 50 people, and closing shopping malls, to mention but a few. On the 20th of March, given the steep growth in the number of people infected with COVID-19 which had already surpassed 400 cases, and the approaching Easter holiday which in Poland is a time of traditional family meetings, the government decided to introduce a state of epidemic. On the 24th of March, further limitations were imposed on gatherings which were limited to a maximum of two people. Exceptions to this were related to families, religious festivities, including masses in the Catholic Church, funerals and marriages (with a maximum of five people), and work places. Moreover, traveling was prohibited with the exception of traveling to your work or home, COVID-19-related activities or other 'necessary everyday activities' (e.g., shopping, visiting the doctor or pharmacy, and also jogging or walking). Importantly, these restrictions, broadened and prolonged several times through the regulations issued by the Minister of Health and Council of Ministers, were considered unconstitutional by the opposition and many experts and civil society organizations. In their opinion, such restrictions could only be imposed within the extraordinary measures

[1] A. Kublik, Jak rząd od 9 stycznia walczył z koronawirusem. *Gazeta Wyborcza*, 19/03/2020.

[2] Special act anticipating coronavirus outbreak passed in Polish parliament. *Notes from Poland*, 3/03/2020.

stipulated in the Constitution (i.e., state of emergency or state of natural disaster). However, due to the presidential elections scheduled for the 10th of May, the government decided not to use any constitutionally regulated, extraordinary measures, as this would delay the elections until 90 days after such a state was lifted. The ruling party did not want any delays, being fully aware that any unexpected consequences of the pandemic could undermine Duda's chances for re-election. All the opposition parties, including Confederation, PO, and PSL, were consistently and unanimously claiming that solutions adopted by PiS were unconstitutional and represented PiS as a party striving for power at any price. On the other hand, PiS and Duda enjoyed extraordinary support from the public media, resorting to polarizing discourse and portraying their opponents as a threat to national identity and interests.

It is very difficult to distinguish the third phase of the government's response to the pandemic based on the death toll or the daily number of people infected which stayed at approximately same level during entire period under consideration. Strict precautionary measures introduced initially by the government kept the number of infections and the death toll at a relatively low level, but on the other hand they led to a considerable social backlash, widespread exhaustion with the restrictions and a growing suspicion that the risks of COVID-19 were exaggerated. This popular feeling was further strengthened by the government's decision, to lift a number of restrictions just after Easter. The government, unable to keep the country locked-down, announced its four-stage plan on April 16th. That decision, unrelated to the number of infections which still oscillated between 250 and 500 (with occasional peaks), only strengthened those suspicions and contributed to a more relaxed approach to the existing limitations among the general public. The most recent changes included lifting the obligation to cover the mouth and nose in some public places (since May 30th) or opening gyms or swimming pools (from June 6th). Accordingly, in Poland, there was no clear mitigation of contagion phase which could be distinguished on the basis of the clear and visible drop of the number of daily cases of infection. Such state of affairs was exploited by PO and PSL and their candidates to emphasize the incumbent's inability to effectively deal with the crisis. The debate was fuelled in May by the revelations regarding the purchase of defective and overpriced medical equipment by Health Minister, Szumowski (Fig. 1 and Table 2).

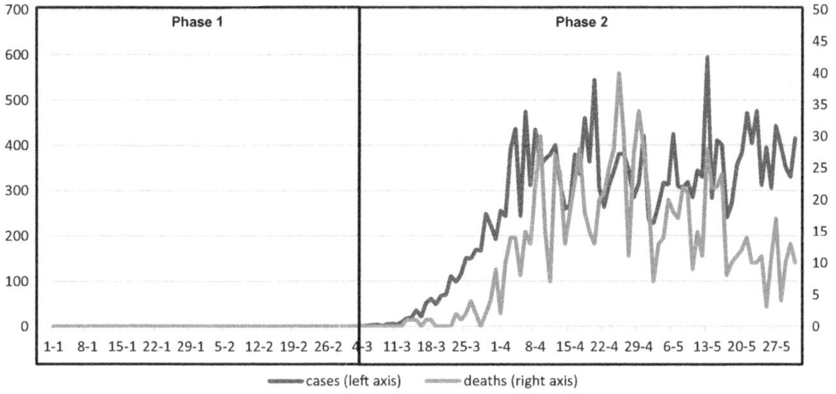

Fig. 1 Daily death toll and new cases in Poland (*Source* European Centre for Disease Prevention and Control. Phase 1: pre-COVID-19; Phase 2: spread and containment measures)

Table 2 COVID-19 pandemic in Poland by June 10, 2020

Cases	27,842
Total deaths	1206
Total recovered	13,411
Cases per 1 million	736
Deaths per 1 million	32

Source www.worldometers.info/coronavirus/ (update 10/6/2020)

4 Populist Discourse at the Time of COVID-19

Political discourse during the COVID-19 pandemic in Poland has been determined by two contextual factors. The first was the difference in institutional position. PiS, as a major government party, was expected to design and implement an efficient response to the spread of the virus. Confederation, the smallest party in parliament, with no prospects of changing its place as the opposition in the nearest future, had more room for radical criticism. The second factor was the struggle between PiS and the rest of the parties over the date of the presidential election, which coincided with or even overshadowed any debate on COVID-19.

The ruling party attempted to use the discourse about COVID-19 to strengthen support for PiS, which in turn was intended to produce public support for Duda. The discursive construction of *the people* was based on references to the nation, Poles, or the citizens. Particularly, in the first two phases, PiS deliberately withdrew the antagonistic aspects of its discourse, emphasizing the necessity to keep national unity. The Prime Minister Mateusz Morawiecki referred to the topos of the national history: '*The coronavirus threat is a matter beyond all divisions – at this moment political disputes have no meaning and I will categorically stop all such narratives. In the face of the coronavirus, Polish society should be and is one. […] Let us remember that the history of Poland teaches us one thing – when we are divided, we are vulnerable to external threats, but when united in a common fight, we have always emerged victorious from all the trials we have been faced with as a nation*' (Morawiecki Facebook page, 11/03/20). Moreover, the discourse on COVID-19 provided an opportunity to bolster national pride through permanent references to other countries, particularly in Europe. Poland was represented not only as able to help Italy in its critical situation, but as an example for other states: '*Today, Poland is at the absolute top of the world when it comes to the speed and efficiency of decisions. We prefer to prevent than cure. […] Economic powers such as the United Kingdom, Germany and the United States have followed the path we have set out*' (Morawiecki Facebook page, 24/03/20). References to the people and Poland were used to portray the government as an advocate of the people, listening to its opinions, responding to their problems, and making proper decisions. Unsurprisingly, such references were used many times to legitimize a government package of economic measures known as the Anti-Crisis Shield.

As regards Confederation, although the party decided to moderate its image and resigned from the most controversial forms of *othering*, its oppositional status was expressed through unrelenting anti-elitism. Accordingly, the people were mainly represented as victims of inadvertently or deliberately incorrect decisions made by the elites. The people's health was neglected by PiS pushing toward the elections despite the pandemic: '*Security and human life is of little importance to them, as is equality of citizens before the law, all that matters to them is political interest and election victory, at any cost*' (Confederation Facebook page, 6/04/20). According to Confederation, the people's needs and interests were fully disregarded by the elites conspiring over the people's heads. One notable example of this conspiracy was the government's anti-crisis' measures derided as '*a lifebuoy made of concrete*' (in Polish, this expression denotes apparent help which in practice makes the situation of the receiver even more difficult – AL) and a '*bureaucratic catastrophe*' (Confederation Facebook page, 1/04/20).

The simultaneous occurrence of the pandemic and the elections attenuated the willingness of PiS to resort to anti-elitism. Contrary to the previous 2019 elections, PiS initially strived to moderate its image to avoid being perceived as focusing merely on political matters instead of existential health-related issues. Consequently, in the first two phases, PiS suspended its criticism of the elites. This changed with the growing tension over PiS' reluctance to delay the elections coupled with the fact that the liberal party, Civic Platform (PO), replaced its presidential candidate Małgorzata Kidawa-Błońska with the mayor of Warsaw, Rafał Trzaskowski. Trzaskowski could easily be targeted as part of the urban, well educated, and liberal elite. Anti-elitism was employed not only by the incumbent President Duda, but also by the Prime Minister Morawiecki: '*Is Poland supposed to be the Poland of elites [...] who want to serve foreigners in a comprador manner, or is it supposed to be the Poland of all Poles, even those who were forgotten, left on the margins of the transformation process? For us, the answer is clear*'.[3] Another line of criticism was directed against the EU, accused of showing a lack of interest and having a slow response to the COVID-19 pandemic. These fallacious assumptions were subsequently used to construct an argument supporting the concept that a loose network of nation-states ('The Europe of the fatherlands') would be more suited to dealing with the crisis.[4]

Contrary to PiS, the discourse of Confederation was entirely based on the antagonistic representation of the elite, the system, and the establishment, frequently referring to the other parliamentary parties as 'the gang of four.' Confederation attempted to pit the people against the elites by exploiting the health crisis and PiS' efforts not to postpone the elections. According to Confederation, the other parties and their candidates were only interested in petty political games. They ignored the real problems of the people, were unwilling to represent their interests, and used the COVID-19 pandemic to strengthen their power and pursue their own narrow interests. Their discursive construction of the crisis was based on emotionally charged labels and arguments, frequently resorting to

[3] M. Morawiecki, Sprawozdanie Stenograficzne z 12. posiedzenia Sejmu Rzeczypospolitej Polskiej w dniu 4 czerwca 2020 r.

[4] A. Mierzyńska, Unia bierna wobec koronawirusa? Manipulacje i ignorancja wiceministra Kowalskiego, *OKO Press*, 17/04/2020.

extremely negative blame attributions. Sometimes Confederation went as far as to imply the betrayal of the people by the elites: 'Companies go bankrupt, workers are laid off, millions of Poles worry about their future, and POPiS (acronym for PO and PiS, suggesting their collusion – AL) ignores this and instead of helping citizens in this difficult time, they turn their backs on entrepreneurs and workers, condemning them to difficult months and years ahead. Is this still the Polish government?!' (Confederation Facebook Profile, 1/04/20). Interestingly, in their attempts to moderate the image of the party, they portrayed the elites as careless, ignorant, and provoking panic, in contrast to Confederation who are sensible, meritocratic, and focused on people's interests instead of power games.

Accordingly, contrary to previous electoral campaigns, references to the 'others' were virtually non-existent in Confederation's discourse. The same applied to PiS in the first two phases of the crisis. In the third phase, however, when confronted with Trzaskowski who was known for supporting the rights of the LGBT community, Duda decided to present himself as a defender of traditional family values through attacks on the LGBT community. Interestingly, the aim of PiS to protect Polish families from COVID-19 was occasionally articulated together with homophobic discourse defining LGBT as an 'ideology' that was 'worse than communism'.[5]

5 The Politicization of COVID-19 Issue by Populists

The context of the electoral campaign and PiS' reluctance to delay the elections has contributed to the rapid politicization of the issue by the opposition. Initially, PiS was interested in securing the broadest support and legitimacy necessary to successfully implement radical pre-emptive measures and build an image of competence and professionalism in dealing with the epidemic. As time went on, they increasingly resorted to polarization, a politics of fear and adoption of the law in a majoritarian fashion.

[5] A. Szczęśniak, Świat patrzy na homofoba Andrzeja Dudę i puka się w czoło. Raport z kampanii, *OKO Press*, 14/06/2020.

Confederation's strategy was much more ambiguous. On the one hand, they were interested in shaking off their image as an ideologically driven party of radicals and eccentrics and win the electorate over as a group with a perfectly normal, mainstream, right-wing identity. On the other hand, as the main rival of PiS on the right, they aimed at attacking the government and president. Consequently, the strategy was based on calculated ambivalence where rhetorical appeals to sensibility, common sense, and constructive proposals on how to combat the epidemic were accompanied by a fierce criticism of the incumbents.

In the *emergence phase*, the governing PiS strived to depoliticize the issue of the pandemic by emphasizing its own efforts to manage the situation, assuring the public that Poland is fully prepared to face COVID-19, providing detailed information about what steps have been and will be taken, and appealing to political parties for national unity: '*Calm and professionalism – this is what we need the most today. So let's not get caught up in attempts to politicize this problem. [...] As Prime Minister, I will not allow the health of Poles to be a matter of political games!*' (Morawiecki Facebook page, 2/03/20). Significantly, attempts to take the issue of the pandemic off the political agenda were coupled with messages highlighting the problem of fake news about COVID-19 and how it might provoke panic in society. However, already at this phase, PiS and President Duda attempted to use the health crisis as an opportunity to present the incumbent president as a leader in the battle against the virus.

Although Confederation rejected the special act on COVID-19 adopted in the emergence phase, it portrayed itself as a meritocratic party, willing to debate the technical issues related to the threat of COVID-19, and refraining from blame games. During a special session of parliament, its presidential candidate, Bosak, was even admonishing the oppositional PO for spreading conspiracy theories. In line with its calculated strategy of ambivalence, the group took an even more radical stance on Facebook by attacking the parliamentarians for conspiring against society and using the threat of COVID-19 as an opportunity to limit civic freedom and undermine the free market (Confederation Facebook page, 1/04/20).

The *confrontation phase* started on March 28th, triggered by PiS' attempts to hold the elections despite serious doubts about its safety. PiS decided to push through amendments to the electoral law which would allow it to organize elections while still being able to refute accusations of exposing Poles to danger. The amendment, part of the Anti-Crisis Shield, would allow people over 60 and those in quarantine or self-isolation to use postal voting. Importantly, the amendment infringed on the ruling of the Constitutional Tribunal according to which significant changes to the electoral law should be made at least six months before elections are called.[6] In its efforts to secure the re-election of its candidate before the expected economic consequences of the lockdown affected public support for Duda, PiS went a step further. On the 6th of April, the Sejm (the lower chamber of the Polish parliament) adopted a bill that would allow people to vote in the May election exclusively by postal vote. In the meantime, PiS politicians were threatening that the consequences of not having an election would be dire and accused oppositional parties of wreaking havoc and breaking democratic rules. As Duda put it: '*If we don't elect the President, the country will plunge into chaos.*'[7] The critical comments and legal response of EU officials and institutions were met with similarly inimical reactions, with the EU being accused of interfering with internal democratic processes.[8] Ultimately, due to the split in the governing coalition, the bill was not approved. Subsequently, the Polish parliament adopted a new electoral law that allowed Poles to either vote traditionally or through postal voting. Moreover, the first round was rescheduled for the 28th of June, which opened a new and even more polarized phase of the campaign. The parliamentary debate over the law provided the oppositional parties the opportunity to criticize PiS for the legal chaos and alleged willingness to introduce authoritarian system.

During the confrontation phase, Confederation consistently demanded the delay of the presidential elections, aware that a drop in the public opinion polls for Duda might easily translate into support for their own presidential candidate. Consequently, Bosak was among the first to announce the claim: '*Let's postpone the election, let's not use the pandemic to make politics! [...] Calling millions of Poles to polling stations during the #coronavirus pandemic is a recipe for mass infections and deaths*' (Confederation Facebook page, 15/03/20). Moreover, the strict epidemic measures and a difficult economic situation opened a discursive window of opportunity for Confederation's radically libertarian agenda. Initially, it politicized the crisis by criticizing PiS' response to COVID-19

[6] D. Tilles, changes to electoral code paving way for May presidential elections passed by Polish parliament, *Notes from Poland*, 28/03/2020.

[7] A. Duda, Bez wyborów kraj będzie w chaosie, *Gazeta Polska*, 22/04/2020.

[8] M. Pankowska, Diagnoza Kaczyńskiego: chce słabszej Unii, bo silna Europa stoi mu na przeszkodzie, *OKO Press*, 16/04/2020.

as too slow and then went on to reveal the weaknesses and oppressiveness of the allegedly socialist state built by PiS as too restrictive toward ordinary citizens and overly bureaucratic toward small entrepreneurs.

The *managing phase* was inextricably linked to previous phases. PiS quite rapidly started to blame the opposition for trying to destabilize the country and undermine democracy, and boasted of its efforts to manage the economic ramifications of the health crisis. The measures implemented by the four editions of the 'Anti-Crisis Shield' were key. The most important of these included the temporary exemption of micro-entrepreneurs and the self-employed from obligatory monthly social security payments, financial benefits for the self-employed, subsidies for employees' wages, and enabling CIT and PIT taxpayers who bore the negative consequences of COVID-19 to deduct the loss incurred in 2020 from operating income generated in 2019. Confederation, striving to present itself as a constructive opposition during parliamentary sessions and through social media communication, consistently listed a number of measures which should have been taken by the government and insisted their demands be taken into account by the governing majority. Moreover, in line with its libertarian agenda, Confederation demanded an immediate lift of lockdown-related restrictions, huge tax reductions for entrepreneurs, and the compensation of salaries not paid by companies whose operations had been stopped by the government.

6 Conclusion

The COVID-19 crisis had a significant impact on the strategies undertaken by PiS during the presidential campaign. Initially, given the weakness of the original Civic Platform candidate and the high level of public support for the incumbent Duda, PiS had reason to believe that Duda was on track for an inevitable landslide victory. The outbreak of the epidemic opened a public discussion on the possibility of delaying the elections and prompted PiS to take unconstitutional measures to prevent such a scenario. The party feared the unforeseen consequences of the crisis, which could negatively affect Duda's chances of re-election. However, the crisis also opened a window of opportunity for the governing camp. In the first phase, preceding the outbreak of the crisis, PiS strived for depoliticization to strengthen the 'rally effect,' with worried citizens united behind government calls for national unity. In addition, restrictive measures against the epidemic created an uneven political struggle, evidently strengthening the incumbent president. This, however, entailed fierce political antagonisms in the subsequent phases, strong politicization of the dispute, and the use of all possible means to push through the elections as scheduled. As a result, PiS could now be criticized as a party that wanted to use the epidemic for political purposes, and the issue of postponing the elections revealed divisions in the United Right coalition power camp.

As for Confederation, the crisis did not fundamentally affect its strategy for becoming more mainstream. The group used the pandemic to build the image of a competent and moderate actor able to offer concrete policy solutions. In addition, the restrictions of the crisis created an opportunity for the libertarian message of the Confederation. Moreover, the Confederation skilfully used its calculated ambivalence to secure the support of its radical electorate. With regard to the polls, in the period under consideration, there was a clear and steady increase in support for both Law and Justice and Duda. During the containment phase, Duda even saw his poll rating exceed 56%. Finally, the crisis did not significantly improve the social support for Confederation, which oscillated between 6 and 9%.[9] The first round of elections held on June 28 confirmed the electoral support for Bosak and his party, providing him 6.78% of the votes. The prolonged, exhaustive campaign, legally doubtful (to say the least) decisions of PiS and scandals over medical equipment purchases coupled with the dynamic campaign of the new PO candidate Trzaskowski contributed to the relatively weak result of Duda. Although he was able to secure 43.5% of the votes in a first round of elections and Trzaskowski only 30.46%, in a second-round run-off he won only with a narrow margin of 51% to 49% for Trzaskowski.

References

Lipiński, A. (2016). *Prawica na polskiej scenie politycznej. Historia, organizacja, tożsamość*. Warszawa: Elipsa.

Moffitt, B. (2015). How to Perform Crisis: A Model for Understanding the Key Role of Crisis in Contemporary Populism. *Government and Opposition, 50*(2), 189–217.

Pankowski, R. (2011). *The Populist Radical Right in Poland: The Patriots*. London: Routledge.

[9] Source: https://www.politico.eu/europe-poll-of-polls/poland/.

Sikk, A. (2012). Newness as a Winning Formula for New Political Parties. *Party Politics, 18*(4), 465–486.

Stanley, B., & Cześnik, M. (2019). Populism in Poland (67–87). In D. Stockemer (Ed.), *Populism Around the World: A Comparative Perspective.* Cham: Springer.

Stone, D. A. (1989). Causal Stories and the Formation of Policy Agendas. *Political Science Quarterly, 104*(2), 281–300.

CHAPTER 10

Between Mitigation and Dramatization: The Effect of the COVID-19 Crisis on Populists' Discourses and Strategies

Giuliano Bobba and Nicolas Hubé

It is generally believed that populists benefit from crisis situations. However, the COVID-19 health crisis is an unconventional event that, at the time of writing this conclusion, is far from being under control. The general research question addressed by this book relates to the possibility that populists in Europe are profiting from a peculiar crisis such as COVID-19, gaining centrality in the political field and/or using the crisis to push forward new opposition lines (RQ1). A second, related, question

G. Bobba (✉)
Department of Cultures, Politics and Society—Collegio Carlo Alberto, University of Turin, Turin, Italy
e-mail: giuliano.bobba@unito.it

N. Hubé
Centre for Research on Mediations (CREM), University of Lorraine, Metz, France
e-mail: nicolas.hube@univ-lorraine.fr

G. Bobba and N. Hubé (eds.), *Populism and the Politicization of the COVID-19 Crisis in Europe*,
https://doi.org/10.1007/978-3-030-66011-6_10

has tried to pinpoint whether populists reacted in a similar way across countries or whether they adapted their response according to their institutional role—in power or not (RQ2). Findings show that while populists have tried to take advantage of the crisis situation, the impossibility of taking ownership of COVID-19 has made benefits more difficult to gain and dependent on the institutional role held.

1 Who Has Benefited from the Crisis? Citizens' Support, Public Relevance, and Windows of Opportunity

There is a priori no political purpose to, or direct responsibility for the origin of the pandemic. Contrary to previous European crises (i.e. financial and migrant), the causes are accidental and determined by unintended and unguided shocks. These accidents are difficult to politicize since they are caused by 'events beyond human control'. For this issue, the process of politicization is therefore more complex, since causal attribution of responsibility is not always possible and unambiguous (Stone 1989). In addition, governments have tried to manage the COVID-19 crisis as a non-political and science-based task, steering the problem away from intentional cause and pushing it towards the realm of nature. Public awareness of the problem in a 'high-choice media environment' (Van Aelst et al. 2017) has made citizens highly informed and given them a means of scanning the evolution of the pandemic in the same way as governments. Transparency and (rational) explanations of governmental decisions have thus been demanded loudly by public opinion throughout Europe.

In the eight European cases analysed in this book, it has been a fact that governments have taken similar health-policy decisions, regardless of their liberal, conservative or populist positioning and the relatively high or low impact of COVID-19.

Of course, there have been some variations in the responses: during the early days of the pandemic, Boris Johnson claimed to be in favour to herd immunity in the UK; Spain, Italy and France experienced a strict lockdown, while Germany, the Czech Republic, Poland and Hungary had lighter forms of movement restrictions and control. These differences, however, have been more a matter of variations by degrees than of the nature of the measures taken. Everywhere, the health emergency

Table 1 Consequences of the COVID-19 crisis on populist parties' performance

	COVID-19 impact	*Populists' role*	*Crisis consequences*
UK	High	Brexit Party: in opposition	Decreasing political relevance and support in the polls
Spain	High	Podemos: in power	Stable institutional relevance and decreasing support in the polls and in local elections
		Vox: in opposition	Increasing institutional relevance and increasing support in the polls and in local elections
Italy	High	M5S: in power	Increasing institutional relevance and stable support in the polls
		Lega: in opposition	Decreasing political relevance and support in the polls
France	High	RN: in opposition	Stable institutional relevance and support in the polls and in local elections
		LFI: in opposition	Stable institutional relevance and decreasing support during the local elections
Germany	Medium	AfD: in opposition	Stable institutional relevance and support in the polls.
Hungary	Medium	Fidesz: in power	Stable and high levels of public support and political centrality
Poland	Low	PiS: in power	Stable institutional relevance and slight decrease in support in the presidential elections
		Konfederacja: in opposition	Stable institutional relevance and public support
Czech Republic	Low	ANO: in power	Stable and high levels of public support and political centrality
		KSČM: external support	Stable levels of public support and institutional political relevance
		SPD: in opposition	

has been the highest priority of the State, allowing the adoption of exceptional temporary measures (such as state of emergency). Only several weeks after the outbreak in Wuhan and its appearance in Europe, it was realized that warnings from the World Health Organization (WHO) and the European Centre for Disease Prevention and Control (ECDPC) had to be taken seriously. Each government thus appointed a scientific and medical committee upon which to rely for the most important decisions. In the same vein, the Europeanization of the crisis has also meant that the timetable for policy decisions has been fairly similar between countries. Because the pandemic arrived there some weeks earlier than elsewhere, Italy showed other European countries how to act, allowing them to structure their health-policy solutions accordingly. Nevertheless, despite this Europeanization of the crisis, responses were not coordinated at the EU level. On the contrary, they can be more clearly interpreted in the light of the political balance of each country.

While crises can usually serve as a window of opportunity for populist parties to maintain a high degree of polarization in debates and crisis-handling action (Moffitt 2015), the COVID-19 pandemic generated a completely different and new context. The suddenness of this external crisis has produced different outcomes for populists depending on whether they are in power or in opposition. In general, populist parties in power have exploited this critical situation to foster their political centrality and legitimacy. M5S in Italy, Podemos in Spain, PiS in Poland, Fidesz in Hungary and ANO in the Czech Republic saw this as an opportunity to show their ability to take care of the people even during a pandemic. In countries where populists are firmly in power and the COVID-19 impact has been low (Hungary, Poland and the Czech Republic), populist leaders have used the rhetoric of the outstanding leader who 'provides direction' to his people (Weyland 2017) through the evocation of threat and reassurance (Edelman 1977). On the contrary, where populist parties are in a coalition government (i.e. PODEMOS and M5S), populist stances have been softened by governmental solidarity and the necessity to justify these extraordinary decisions. In other words, in contrast to the evidence that emerged previously (Albertazzi and McDonnell 2015; Pappas 2019), the strategy of populists in power has been quite the reverse of that adopted in normal situations: forced to deal with a non-controversial issue, they have tried to depoliticize the issue and to reduce the level of polarization around it.

For populist parties in opposition, the use of their classical tactics during the pandemic crisis has been certainly complicated. Since the crisis has pervaded every aspect of public and private life, to 'perform and spread a sense of crisis' (Moffitt 2015) has been virtually impossible. The main strategy that has generally succeeded has been an insistence on the need to overcome the health crisis by the nation as a whole. The emergence and success of divisive and polarizing counter-arguments have not only been difficult to achieve but also potentially damaging in terms of image and reputation for populist parties. This explains why, with a few exceptions (i.e. the Brexit Party criticizing the lockdown), all the opposition populist parties included in this study voted for the emergency measures during phase 2. Hindered by the discourse of national unity that could have made their criticisms perceived as inappropriate, French populists, for example, were forced to shift the focus of their critique using the most legitimate political tool at their disposal: legislative activities at a time when parliament was in semi-lockdown.

Only after several weeks and the mitigation of the contagion (phase 3) were populist parties able to get back to their key arguments, especially those against the national and supranational elite as well as migrants. The crisis has led to the radicalization of discourse for the Brexit Party, Vox and Konfederacja, acting as a trigger for a more intense campaign against the 'enemies of the people'. The AfD, instead, has been hindered by more radical stances of the extra-parliamentary opposition (APO). Finally, in other countries—like Italy, France or the SPD in the Czech Republic—populist parties in opposition have resumed their classical stances, updating their discursive repertoire to the new COVID-19 age.

To sum up, it is hard to identify a single populist pattern during the pandemic. In general, it seems that the populists have not substantially benefited, nor substantially lost out, from the COVID-19 crisis: governing populist parties have maintained or slightly increased their centrality and public support, whereas opposition parties have remained stable or have seen their positions slightly worsen. A possible explanation is that policy options converged towards a few shared solutions, especially in phases 1 and 2. This means that populist and non-populist parties have often voted together, despite the rhetoric from both sides describing the two types of party as irreconcilable. The need to overcome the crisis appears, therefore, to have left the situation apparently unchanged in the short term. However, it might be worth exploring what will happen in the medium term. Although, as mentioned earlier, in phase 3 some populist actors returned to their pre-crisis rhetoric, the COVID-19 pandemic has introduced two new elements that could point to certain consequences in the coming months. On the one hand, it has shown that populist parties, far from being a democratic aberration, are political actors in all respects that can contribute to finding solutions and implementing policies. On the other hand, it has also shown that the post-COVID-19 age could offer new opportunities in terms of alliances and policy repositioning—such as the role of science or strengthening the health system—between populist and non-populist parties (Table 1).

2 The Changing Relevance of the Key Elements of Populism in the Light of (De)Politicization of the COVID-19 Issue

While populists have not really benefited from the crisis, they have had to face it like all the other political players and adapt their discourse to this unprecedented situation, outside the usual framework of political competition. In particular, as already mentioned, COVID-19 initially had the effect of restraining any form of radical opposition to the policy responses to be implemented, at least in the European Union. During the first month of the crisis, with very few exceptions (i.e. some claims by the Brexit Party, the AfD and the Lega), the pandemic was not a subject of political confrontation. Other 'normal' issues were at stake within national debates, including, for example, strikes and local elections in France. Suddenly, from the beginning of the *confrontation phase* onwards (end of February-beginning of March), COVID-19 became the overwhelming subject, crowding out all other issues at stake on the EU and national political agenda. The general opinion—both public and political—was consensual: there is an urgent need to act to protect the population from the pandemic.

One of the aims of this book was to identify how populists have adapted their discourse to the pandemic crisis (RQ1a). As regards the action of ***naming*** (Felstiner et al. 1980), all the political actors (both populist and otherwise, in power or in opposition) moved rapidly from minimizing the problem as a minor form of flu or a Chinese disease to admitting the seriousness of the health emergency, without any other form of intermediate categorization. No symbolic struggle or political opposition to its naming was noted from March to June: the COVID-19 pandemic was recognized in all countries and by all main political parties as a scientific challenge and a relevant issue to be solved.

As a result of the urgency of finding a response, it is noteworthy that both *blaming* and *claiming* actions have been concomitant and quite fluctuating (Katsambekis and Stavrakakis 2020). Prevented from using the appeal to the people as an original and effective argument, during the *confrontation* and *managing* phases, populists emphasized the other two key elements—anti-elitism and exclusionism. Depending on the national political game, criticism of a slow and uncoordinated EU-elite responsiveness has taken different forms: in the United Kingdom, for example, Nigel Farage saw the crisis as an opportunity to call for a no-deal Brexit; in Italy, meanwhile, after years of austerity, the arguments were framed around the European Stability Mechanism (ESM) blamed as a tool used to limit the economic autonomy of the country. Not all anti-elite claims are, however, necessarily specific to populists. There can be much more wide-ranging issues at stake at the national level. For instance, criticism of the unpreparedness of the French government was endorsed by the entire political and media spectrum; similarly, worries about European austerity measures are widely shared in Italy. A second blaming theme concerned the handling of migration issues. While in the UK, Germany, Poland, Hungary, the Czech Republic and Spain this included the request to close borders to reduce the risk of contagion from abroad, in France and Italy the two right-wing populist leaders, Marine Le Pen and Matteo Salvini, accused governments of taking care of migrants instead of focusing only on nationals.

This book also found evidence that right-wing and left-wing populist parties have reacted in a very different way to the challenge of the COVID-19 crisis. On the one hand, right-wing populism has identified new lines of conflict: an intensification of the emphasis on nationalism (and neo-natalism) and the (resulting) opposition of 'we, the national people', not only against the EU but also against the other member States. These findings confirm that right-wing populism and Euroscepticism are reinforcing each other (Conti 2018; Rooduijn and van Kessel 2019). On the other hand, it is evident that left-wing parties (Podemos, LFI and to a certain extent M5S) are not using this kind of discourse. During the crisis, they were more focused on denouncing the lack of public investment in the national healthcare system and the disastrous consequences of years of EU neoliberalism.

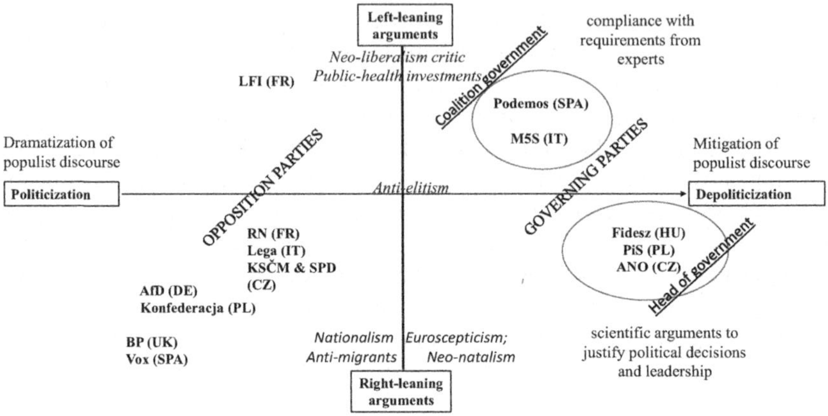

Fig. 1 Map of European populist discourse faced with the COVID-19 crisis

Country-specific chapters also offer relevant findings regarding the politicization of COVID-19 issues by populist parties (RQ1b). Similarly to Euroscepticism (Sitter 2001; Hubé 2013), the way populists in power and populists in opposition have faced COVID-19 emphasizes the importance of the institutional role in party behaviour (RQ2). Being (or not being) in power structures partisan discourse. Politicization strategies may be placed on a continuum line ranging from complete politicization to complete depoliticization, structured around the party's position in the national institutional framework. The combination of politicization line with left-right positioning provides a relational map of the different arguments and reactions of populists in the eight countries analysed (Fig. 1).[1]

On the one hand, opposition parties tried to politicize the pandemic, but they only partly succeeded, in phase 3, mainly focusing on the management of the pandemic and blaming the ruling parties. No populist party has attempted to politicize the pandemic outbreak as, for example, Donald Trump did by questioning the origin of the virus. The institutional position has seemed to play a major role in this politicization process. The most marginal parties (i.e. the Brexit Party, Vox, AfD and

[1] The map provides a qualitative classification of different party positions based on the evidence that emerged from the national chapters.

Konfederacja) have clearly radicalized their discourse based on nationalist, protectionist and neo-natalist agendas. The opposition parties aspiring to govern—such as RN, LFI and Lega—have been much more cautious, mainly focusing on alleged governmental incompetence.

On the other hand, governmental parties have tried to depoliticize the crisis using technical and scientific arguments, following the recommendations of national experts. For them, the crisis has been an excellent chance to show their political competence, managerial abilities and dedication to the people. The most typical case here is undoubtedly the Czech Republic, whose Prime Minister, Andrej Babiš, has stressed his ability to govern the country in this situation as successfully as he managed his companies in the past. Again, a difference seems to emerge between left-wing and right-wing populists in power. Podemos in Spain and M5S in Italy, as members of coalition governments, have based their political action on the advice of the technical-scientific committee, denouncing the need for more public investment in health care. At the opposite end of the spectrum, right-wing populists in power in Poland, Hungary and the Czech Republic have mainly used scientific arguments to justify their political decisions, emphasizing their leader's ability to make informed decisions solely on the basis of the authority of their political leadership.

A clear pattern of politicization of the COVID-19 crisis by populist political parties in Europe can thus be observed. The institutional position of the party in the national political game affects the way populists have addressed the issues, ranging from mitigation of populist discourse (populists in power) to its dramatization (populists in opposition).

It is worth noting that this pattern based on the institutional role works for the cases analysed here but does not include a further situation that everyone has heard of: some leaders in power have rejected the scientific evidence on the virus and have used the dispute between politicians and scientists to justify political decisions (Katsambekis and Stavrakakis 2020). Aside from some initial (and careless) statements by Boris Johnson and some comments between Farage and Trump, in Europe this kind of populist governmental style seems to be absent. It is also somewhat surprising that no leaders analysed here have given credit to or supported the conspiracy theories that are usually an integral part of populist strategy (Bergmann 2018). In France, the debate around the chloroquine (HCQ) issue could have been endorsed by populist leaders, while in fact all the main French political actors distanced themselves from this scientific controversy when the debate became too sticky. Similarly, in Italy, both

M5S and Lega—close to the No-Vax movement in recent years—have not argued against big pharma companies or stirred any controversy against the scientific world. The number of intensive care patients and the death toll has likely discouraged European populist leaders from resorting to this kind of argumentation.

3 Crises as a Catalyst for Change, Populists as Entrepreneurs of Crises

The literature has interpreted crises as opportunities for change (see Chapter 1). A crisis occurs when systemic contradictions are politically exploited and publicly perceived as such (Hay 1999). Populists are generally considered to benefit from a crisis: they play an active role as crisis facilitators by pushing problematic situations towards a crisis at both the political and communicative levels (Moffitt 2015). The success of populism is then often interpreted as the result of an external crisis (economic, financial, political, migrant, traditional values), questioning the problem-solving rationality with respect to a certain issue. Populists take advantage of this fuzziness to propose their clear and popular policy solutions. This general pattern seems not to work when applied to the COVID-19 crisis. As already mentioned, the peculiar nature of the crisis, as well as the implementation of similar policy solutions across all the European States, has virtually prevented populists from gaining centrality in the political field and support from public opinion.

Nevertheless, slightly broadening the analytical perspective and taking into account the relational approach through which parties position themselves in the national political field (Bourdieu 1991), it is noticeable that all populist actors acted as 'crisis entrepreneurs', that is, as someone who identifies, denounces and claims to be the solver of one or more systemic contradictions. As they have been unable to exploit the COVID-19 issue—or able to do so to a limited extent—the populists analysed in this book have focused their actions on the new contradictions emerging from the crisis situation, such as the role of the EU in managing the health problem and the economic recovery plan; the opposition of interests between European States; the unresolved issue of migrant arrivals.

Evidence suggests that populists—in power or in opposition—benefit more from a situation of continual complaint against new contradictions than from the actual outbreak of a crisis (i.e. COVID-19) or, worse still, from a solution to it (i.e. Brexit for the UKIP). In fact, populists are crisis entrepreneurs who strive to fuel a permanent crisis cycle. This is, in fact, the condition that allows them to take full advantage of crises in terms of political centrality and voter support. Of course, as already mentioned, not all crises are the same. Populists take ownership of the contradictions that best suit their Manichean view of society. The quest for this crisis ownership is what feeds the continuous process of *naming*, *blaming*, *claiming* of systemic contradictions that populists implement as a political strategy.

Figure 2 summarizes the permanent crisis cycle fuelled by populists. In a usual situation, the pattern begins with the emergence, triggered by populists, of a political contradiction (1), which becomes publicly recognized as a relevant problem (2) and is exploited by populists (3), who push it towards an actual crisis (4). Populists do not focus on one contradiction at a time; on the contrary, they trigger this cycle for all the

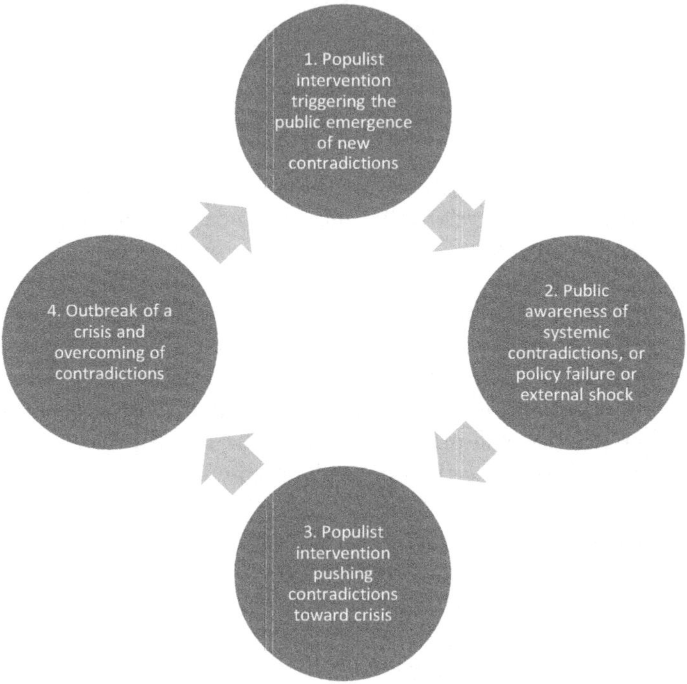

Fig. 2 Permanent crisis cycle fuelled by populists

contradictions they see at a given time. Points 1 to 3 are the moments when populists can benefit the most from the crisis situation, while in point 4, the climax, the contradiction finds a solution or a compromise that weakens the issue.

In external shocks, such as the pandemic outbreak, all political actors suddenly found themselves in point 4, where a crisis had broken out and a solution had to be found. This is the worst condition for populists because citizens perceive problems as real or experience them directly, and so political responses must be rapidly implemented. At these critical junctures, disputes and polarization often leave room for forms of political collaboration or non-hostile, tacit agreement in the name of national solidarity. However, as soon as this state of emergency ends, populists begin to implement the permanent crisis strategy again, fostering the emergence of new contradictions (point 1). This is exactly what happened in the eight countries analysed in this book between March and June.

In our view, therefore, crises per se do not necessarily benefit populism. It is populists, instead, who fuel a 'permanent crisis cycle' consisting of a continuous quest for 'crisis ownership' around stable or emerging political contradictions. The COVID-19 pandemic is an interesting case for which populists have been unable to achieve this kind of ownership, at least so far.

The health crisis, however, is anything but over, nor under control. On the contrary, after a relatively quiet summer, the second wave of the outbreak seems to be worse than the previous one.

For a few months now, COVID-19 has moved into policy routine and governments are oscillating between economic, public health and preventive policy measures. In the coming months, the COVID-19 crisis will be then 'normalized', becoming the new standard situation in which political struggle will occur and the people will have to live. This normalization of the COVID-19 crisis will probably offer to the opposition parties greater opportunities to politicize the policies implemented by governments and possibly to benefit from the crisis.

However, the factors involved are so numerous—i.e. the actual harshness of the second wave, the economic implications, the discovery of an effective vaccine or medicine—that it is not possible today to outline reliable future scenarios. What we do know, however, is that a political challenge will be played between the parties in power—that risk being worn by the health crisis—and the opposition parties—that could take advantage of the inevitable discontents that the pandemic is generating.

Populists in power and in opposition, therefore, will have to face opposite challenges, the outcome of which will determine the features of the European populism in the post-COVID-19 age.

Turin/Metz, November 2020

References

Albertazzi, D., & McDonnell, D. (2015). *Populists in Power*. Oxon and New-York: Routledge.

Bergmann, E. (2018). *Conspiracy & Populism: The Politics of Misinformation*. Cham: Palgrave Macmillan.

Bourdieu, P. (1991). Political Representation: Elements for a Theory of the Political Field. In P. Bourdieu (Ed.), *Language and Symbolic Power* (pp. 171–202). Harvard: Harvard University Press.

Conti, N. (2018). National Political Elites, the EU, and the Populist Challenge. *Politics, 38*(3), 361–377.

Edelman, M. (1977). *Political Language: Words That Succeed and Policies That Fail*. New York: Academic Press.

Felstiner, W. L. F., Abel, R. L., & Sarat, A. (1980) The Emergence and Transformation of Disputes: Naming, Blaming, Claiming... *Law & Society Review, 15*(3/4), 631–654.

Hay, C. (1999). Crisis and the Structural Transformation of the State: Interrogating the Process of Change. *British Journal of Politics and International Relations, 1*(2), 317–344.

Hubé, N. (2013). France. In N. Conti (Ed.), *Party Attitudes Towards the EU in the Member States: Parties for Europe, Parties Against Europe* (pp. 19–42). London and New York: Routledge.

Katsambekis, G., & Stavrakakis, Y. (Eds.). (2020). Populism and the Pandemic: A Collaborative Report. *POPULISMUS Interventions*, 7.

Moffitt, B. (2015). How to Perform Crisis: A Model for Understanding the Key Role of Crisis in Contemporary Populism. *Government and Opposition, 50*(2), 189–217.

Pappas, T. S. (2019). Populists in Power. *Journal of Democracy, 30*(2), 70–84.

Rooduijn, M., & van Kessel, S. (2019) Populism and Euroskepticism in the European Union. *Oxford Research Encyclopedia of Politics*.

Sitter, N. (2001). The Politics of Opposition and European Integration in Scandinavia: Is Euro-Scepticism a Government-Opposition Dynamic? *West European Politics, 24*(4), 22–39.

Stone, D. (1989). Causal Stories and the Formation of Policy Agendas. *Political Science Quarterly, 104*(2), 281–300.

Van Aelst, P., Strömbäck, J., Aalberg, T., et al. (2017). Political Communication in a High-Choice Media Environment: A Challenge for Democracy? *Annals of the International Communication Association, 41*(1), 3–27.

Weyland, K. (2017). Populism: A Political-Strategic Approach. In C. Rovira Kaltwasser, P. Taggart, P. Ochoa Espejo, & P. Ostiguy (Eds.), *The Oxford Handbook of Populism* (pp. 48–72). Oxford: Oxford University Press.

The manufacturer's authorised representative in the EU is Springer Nature Customer Service Centre GmbH, Europaplatz 3, 69115 Heidelberg, Germany. If you have any concerns regarding our products, please contact ProductSafety@springernature.com

Printed and bound by CPI Group (UK) Ltd, Croydon, CR0 4YY
30/09/2026
02225475-0015